Eat to Beat

TYPE 2 DIABETES

Also by the Hairy Bikers:

Food Tour of Britain
Mums Know Best
Mums Still Know Best
12 Days of Christmas
Perfect Pies
Big Book of Baking
Great Curries
Asian Adventure
Meat Feasts
Chicken and Egg
Mediterranean Adventure
British Classics
One Pot Wonders

Eat to Beat

TYPE 2 DIABETES

Si King & Dave Myers

SEVEN DIALS

First published in Great Britain in 2020 by Seven Dials
an imprint of The Orion Publishing Group Ltd
Carmelite House, 50 Victoria Embankment
London, EC4Y 0DZ
An Hachette UK Company

11 13 15 17 19 20 18 16 14 12

A CIP catalogue record for this book is
available from the British Library.

ISBN (Trade Paperback) 978 1 8418 8407 3
ISBN (eBook) 978 1 8418 8409 7

Photographer: Andrew Hayes-Watkins
Recipe and food consultant: Catherine Phipps
Food stylists: Anna Burges-Lumsden, Lisa Harrison, Mima Sinclair
Editor: Jinny Johnson
Design: Clare Sivell
Proofreader: Elise See Tai
Indexer: Vicki Robinson

Publisher: Vicky Eribo
Project editor: Isabelle Everington

Nutritional information: Fiona Hunter, BSc (Hons) Nutrition, Dip Dietetics

Printed and bound in Great Britain by Clays Ltd, Elcograf S.p.A.

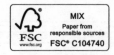

www.orionbooks.co.uk

CONTENTS

FOREWORD
by Professor Roy Taylor
VII

OUR STORY
1

BREAKFAST and BRUNCH
13

SOUPS and SALADS
39

SNACKS and DIPS
73

VEGGIE TREATS
95

HEARTY SUPPERS
139

SIDES and BASICS
189

PUDDINGS and BAKES
215

MEAL PLANNERS
243

INDEX
256

USEFUL ADDRESSES
262

ACKNOWLEDGEMENTS
264

FOREWORD

The Hairy Dieters have a mission to bring sunshine and variety to the notion of 'diet'! People need to eat food. People with type 2 diabetes also need to eat food. In this book, Si and Dave apply their magic to square health needs with varied, enjoyable eating. If you are looking for new and interesting ways to eat, this book is for you.

But what qualifications do the Hairy Bikers have to advise people with type 2 diabetes about what to eat? They parachuted into my life in 2012 to make a TV series about how to lose weight, yet eat well. But they did not just turn up and perform on camera. They rolled up their sleeves and agreed to try and lose the amount of weight that most people with type 2 diabetes *need* to lose. That is around two and a half stone each. And they were to lose this in 12 weeks.

A few days later I received a tentative phone call: did I really mean two and a half stone? Yes, that's right. In Newcastle, we had pioneered the use of low-calorie liquid formula diets to lose weight effectively and reverse type 2 diabetes. But Si and Dave did not want to take the easy route, using packets of a liquid formula diet. They wanted to lose weight while eating real food. So, they worked with my team, especially nutrition expert Professor Ashley Adamson, to devise low-calorie recipes for delicious meals. Then they cooked themselves into losing over three stone each. As qualifications go for writing this book, that is pretty impressive.

In today's world of ready meals and commercially provided fast food, the very basic skill of cooking is in danger of becoming merely an entertainment and not something that everyone can do. So, a book that makes this simple is very timely. The recipes are easy to prepare, and each step is clearly described for the novice. First open the kitchen door!

This book will provide ideas to make healthy cooking more exciting, whether or not you have diabetes. But what is a healthy diet? All the basics of nutrition were worked out in the early nineteenth century. Those basics are, of course, still important – a wide variety of foodstuffs, vitamins, minerals and so on. But in today's overfed environment, a healthy diet is principally one that keeps your weight stable, and similar to your weight in early adult life. The type of foods eaten are important only in that they must satisfy appetite without over-doing the calories. You are not *what* you eat, but rather you are *how much* you eat.

Our detailed studies using special MRI scans have identified the harm caused by carrying around more weight than your own body can cope with. If a person with type 2 diabetes really wants to regain health, losing a substantial amount of weight is the first step. But the most difficult matter is to keep the weight off in the long term. Lifelong. This book should be a stalwart friend in helping you achieve just that.

Roy Taylor
Professor of Medicine and Metabolism
Newcastle University

OUR STORY

Ten years ago, before we started writing our Hairy Dieters cookbooks, we were – to put it bluntly – fat! We had high blood pressure and high cholesterol, Dave was prediabetic and we were heading for problems. But, with great advice and lots of support from healthy eating experts, we turned our lives around and we shed more than six stone between us. Our blood pressure and cholesterol improved and Dave now has his blood sugars under control and has greatly reduced his risk of diabetes. It wasn't always easy – we had to get weighed in our pants on the telly! – but we did it with the help of our great Healthy Dieters' recipes and we felt fantastic.

Creating the recipes for these books was amazing because cooking your food from scratch gives you real control over what you eat. You know exactly what's on your plate and you can limit salt, sugar, fat and so on. That's what makes our Healthy Dieters' recipes ideal for those at risk of, or suffering from, diabetes, so we have made a selection of our recipes to help you lose weight and get diabetes under control.

There are two basic types of diabetes – type 1 and type 2. In this book we are dealing with type 2, the more common form. We know now that for some people type 2 diabetes can be reversed, so you don't need to take medication, and the main route to this is healthy eating and weight loss, plus exercise.

You know us – we're cooks, not medical experts. But it's clear that most people with type 2 diabetes are overweight, and also that being overweight puts you at risk of developing type 2 diabetes. We also know that the right diet is both crucial and helpful, and losing weight is key. So we asked Fiona, our favourite nutrition expert, for some more information and advice.

DAVE: Can you tell us more about diabetes?
FIONA: If you have diabetes your blood sugar levels are too high. With type 1 diabetes the body's immune system destroys the cells that produce insulin. This is a lifelong condition that requires injections to replace the insulin. With type 2 diabetes the body does not produce enough insulin to regulate blood sugar levels and does not react to insulin properly. In both instances, this means that the body is not able to convert sugar to energy. About 90 per cent of people with diabetes in the UK have type 2. Many have to take medication but the condition can be reversed.

There is also a condition called gestational diabetes, which happens to some women in pregnancy. This means that the body does not produce enough insulin for the extra needs of pregnancy, but the condition usually goes away after the baby is born. However, it does indicate a high risk of developing type 2 diabetes in the future.

People may be told that they are at risk of type 2 diabetes, described as prediabetes. This means that their blood sugar is higher than normal but not yet high enough for a diagnosis of diabetes, so the right diet and exercise can help a great deal.

SNACKING

Small but sustaining – that's the message for snacks.
If you have diabetes, you may find that you need a little
something in between meals to stave off those hunger
pangs without sending your blood sugar levels soaring.
Ideally a healthy snack should be low in calories, fat
and sugar but tasty enough to keep you satisfied. Here
are some ideas of snacks that are easy to carry with
you when you're out and about, so you're not tempted
to grab a chocolate bar.

Fresh fruit – such as one apple, satsuma, peach
   or pear
Dried fruit – a few prunes, small box of raisins
Nuts – half a dozen almonds or walnuts (not too many
   as nuts are high in calories)
A rice cake
An oat cake
A few bread sticks
Handful of edamame beans
Hard-boiled egg
Sticks of raw veg such as carrots and cucumber and
   small pot of hummus or **other dips** (see page 78)
Home-made popcorn (see page 92)
Roast chickpeas (see page 90)

SI: So keeping to a weight that is healthy for you is really important. What's the best way to do this?

FIONA: There are all sorts of diets, but in the end the best way to lose weight is to cut calories. If you take in fewer calories, the body has to use its own stores of fat. On average, a man needs about 2,500 calories a day and a woman about 2,000, although this can vary considerably according to body size and activity levels. To lose about a kilo a week you need to cut your calorie intake down to about 1,500–1,800 a day. Obviously you can't maintain this forever, but once you get down to your target weight, just make sure you don't start eating too much again and exceeding your calorie needs.

DAVE: And what about exercise?

FIONA: Yes, burning more calories can help you lose weight, so aim to be physically active every day and combine this with cutting calories. You don't have to go pumping iron in the gym. Find something you enjoy, whether it is sport, dancing, cycling or whatever, and stick with it. The simplest thing is brisk walking, which you can do anywhere and the NHS advice is to do short bursts of at least 10 minutes at a time to raise your heart rate. Try to do 150 minutes a week of moderate intensity activity, such as brisk walking, cycling, dancing or tennis, or 75 minutes of vigorous intensity exercise, such as jogging or running, fast cycling or swimming, or sports like football or hockey. That will help keep your heart healthy as well as help you to lose weight.

It's also important to do some muscle-strengthening exercise a couple of times a week, such as yoga, Pilates, weights or heavy gardening. But if you want to lose weight over a short time, most people do best by not starting a new exercise programme right away, but just by cutting back on food (and alcohol). Then build up activity for the long term.

SI: So now to food. Is it best to eat low-fat products?
FIONA: Fat contains a lot of calories. Gram for gram it contains twice as many calories as protein or carbohydrates (a level teaspoon of butter is 153 calories), so reducing the amount of fat you eat will help you reduce your calorie intake. And it's easy these days, as there are so many low-fat and reduced-fat products in the supermarket. Choose semi-skimmed milk, low-fat yoghurt and reduced-fat crème fraiche and you will cut calories but still enjoy delicious meals.

But be careful. Do have a close look at low-fat products and check the ingredients list, as some are high in sugar. Look out for ingredients such as sucrose, maltose, dextrose, glucose, fructose – these are all sugars. For example, a fruit yoghurt might be low in fat but contain loads of sugar. Choose plain yoghurt instead and add your own fresh fruit if you want.

We all need to eat some fat, as it is important for our bodies, particularly for the brain and nervous system. But we need to make sure it is the right kind of fat. Too much saturated fat can raise cholesterol and make us more at risk of heart disease and strokes. Unsaturated fat can help to keep cholesterol levels healthy and protect the heart.

However, all fat is high in calories so should be eaten in moderation and bear in mind that a reduced-fat label on a product doesn't necessarily mean low-fat. Things like reduced-fat crème fraiche may have less fat than the normal version but may still be quite high in fat, so watch your portion size.

Some foods high in saturated fat

- Butter and lard
- Cheese (especially full-fat cheese)
- Cream and ice cream
- Cakes and biscuits
- Fatty meat, sausages and bacon
- Chocolates
- Crème fraiche (especially full-fat)
- Some types of yoghurt
- Pastry

Foods with unsaturated fat

- Olive oil
- Rapeseed oil
- Avocados
- Nuts and seeds
- Oily fish, such as salmon, mackerel, herring

DAVE: Is it OK to eat fruit if you have type 2 diabetes?
FIONA: People used to worry about this because fruit contains natural sugars, which can affect blood sugar levels. But fruit is also so good for us, so the best advice is to eat a couple of portions of fruit a day and avoid having too much in one go. Be careful with dried fruit, as that contains concentrated sugar, and stick to eating whole fruit rather than drinking fruit juice. Whole fruit contains fibre, which slows down the rate at which you absorb the sugars, but with juice most of the fibre has been removed and you can glug down large amounts in a short time. Think about it: a glass of orange juice might contain the juice – and sugar – from four or five

oranges, but you wouldn't be very likely to eat all those at one sitting. That seductive-looking glass of fruit juice contains a pile of calories.

SI: Can you drink alcohol?
FIONA: Yes, in moderation. But be careful, as alcohol contains plenty of calories – about nine calories a gram – so if you are trying to lose weight cutting down on alcohol will help. Also, people tend to make worse food choices after a few drinks. Willpower dissolves in alcohol! If you do want to drink, stick to the guidelines and have no more than 14 units a week. Don't binge and have this all in one go on a Friday night, and aim to have several alcohol-free days a week. If you drink spirits, make sure you choose sugar-free mixers.

Water is the best drink for staying hydrated. Keep an eye on your pee. If it is a pale straw colour you're doing fine. If it is dark yellow or brown, you're dehydrated and you need to drink more water.

DAVE: Is it best to use sweeteners instead of sugar?
FIONA: Cutting back on the sweet stuff helps keep your blood sugar stable and reduces your calorie intake. Yes, you can use sugar-free sweeteners and they can be a great help, but really the aim should be to train your palate to enjoy food that is less sweet. Try to cut back and learn to enjoy the natural tastes of your food and drinks. If you usually take a couple of spoonfuls of sugar in your tea and coffee, cut down gradually and soon you'll find you are happy without it. If you really can't cope, try sugar-free sweeteners but it is worth persevering, so be patient and give it time.

Sweeteners are fine when you are just adding sweetness and they're very useful in some recipes. Always check the packet for guidelines on how much to use, as they differ. But sometimes, for instance in baking recipes, you need to use proper sugar for texture and volume, but it's best to keep cakes and biscuits to a minimum for an occasional treat.

SI: What about salt?
FIONA: It's important to keep your salt intake down. Salt is associated with high blood pressure, and if you have diabetes you are at an increased risk of heart disease. High blood pressure increases this risk further. Try seasoning with black pepper and allowing your taste buds to adjust to less salty tastes. As with sugar, you can train your taste buds to enjoy foods with less salt. It can take about four weeks but if you stick with it you'll get there.

DAVE: Presumably it's important to have your five a day?
FIONA: Vegetables are our best friends. Make sure you have at least five portions of veg and fruit a day and you'll find they do you good as well as fill you up. That way you'll have less room for unhealthy snacks like sweets and crisps. The concept of 'five insteads a day' says it all – so, for instance, choose an apple for a snack instead of a chocolate biscuit. Find recipes with loads of great veg and feel free to add extras on the side if you need more food. Vegetables, particularly the non-starchy ones, are much lower in calories than meat, dairy products and cereals, and they contain lots of vitamins, minerals and other things called phytochemicals which help to keep you healthy. The more veg you have the better.

VEG ARE OUR BEST FRIENDS

Here are some calorie counts for 80g portions of some of the most popular vegetables – 80g is what counts as one of your five a day and is generally a portion about the same size as a loosely clenched fist. You might be surprised at how few calories vegetables contain – as long as you don't slather them in butter, of course!

Broccoli: 34 calories

Cabbage: 26 calories

Carrots: 34 calories

Cauliflower: 26 calories

Celery: 8 calories

Cherry tomatoes: 20 calories

Courgettes: 16 calories

Green beans: 24 calories

Peas: 76 calories

Red pepper (half): 21 calories

Spinach: 15 calories

Sweetcorn: 52 calories

Compare those calorie counts with those of some popular snacks:

Small bag (25g) of crisps: 132 calories

Oven chips (100g): 157 calories

Small bar (45g) of milk chocolate: 237 calories

1 milk chocolate digestive biscuit: 86 calories

1 sausage roll (100g): 327 calories

SI: What about protein? And meat?

FIONA: You don't have to give up meat if you don't want to, but it's sensible to cut down on red meat and avoid processed meat. Go for fish – particularly oily fish which is good for heart health – and chicken, or choose other forms of protein such as pulses, eggs and nuts. Dairy foods also contain protein but stick to lower-fat versions.

DAVE: And are low-carb diets a good idea?

FIONA: As you know, when you eat carbohydrates the body turns them into glucose, which makes your blood sugar rise. Everyone needs some carbs in their diet, even if you have diabetes, but you do need to choose the right ones. Go for complex carbs that contain plenty of fibre – that's whole grains, vegetables and pulses. These carbs are absorbed slowly by the body, so the sugar is released gradually and is easier to cope with.

Simple carbs, such as cakes, sweets, soft drinks and so on, don't have much fibre, if any, and they contain refined sugars which are absorbed quickly by the body and create sugar surges. They are also high in calories and these are what we call empty calories with no nutritional value – they're not doing you any good at all. Worse still, your body will turn excess sugar into saturated fat, which is bad news.

Some people do well on a low-carb diet but it is important to check with your doctor or dietitian to make sure this is a suitable approach for you.

EATING TO BEAT DIABETES THE HAIRY BIKER WAY

We've got the message and it's simple: start by cooking your own food from scratch, using plenty of vegetables, good high-fibre carbs and some protein. Cut down on salt, sugar and saturated fat, go easy on the alcohol and drink plenty of water. Avoid commercial snacks in between meals – they're usually high in calories. Keep active and you'll soon shed those pounds and improve your health.

It can really help to plan your meals for the week ahead. Write yourself a menu and try to include a wide range of different vegetables and other foods to make sure you get a good balance of nutrients. It's all too easy to get stuck in a rut and buy and cook the same things week after week.

All our recipes are calorie counted to make things easy for you and you might also like to follow the meal planners on pages 243–255 of this book.

A FEW LITTLE NOTES FROM US

We've given calorie counts for our dishes so follow the recipes carefully so you don't change the count. Weigh ingredients and use proper spoons and a measuring jug. We always say how many people a recipe serves, so you don't eat more than your share. Sometimes on packets you will see calories referred to as kilocalories but they are same thing. You might also see figures in kilojoules, which is a different way of measuring the energy in food. These figures will be larger but we are just dealing with calories (kilocalories) in this book so no need to worry about kilojoules.

We mention spray oil in quite a few recipes, as this is an easy way of reducing the amount of oil you use. Buy the most natural kind you can find and spritz it lightly. If you don't want to use spray oil, just brush on a small amount of oil with a pastry brush.

Peel onions, garlic and all other vegetables and fruit unless otherwise specified.

Use free-range eggs and free-range chicken whenever possible. Whatever you're cooking, it always pays to buy the best and freshest seasonal ingredients you can afford. We reckon that 95 per cent of good cooking is good shopping – great ingredients need less fussing with.

We haven't listed salt in most of the recipes because it is best to cut it out. Stick to black pepper and lots of lovely herbs instead.

If you're really organised you might have some of your own home-made stock in your freezer and you'll find our recipes for vegetable stock and chicken stock in this book. Otherwise, it's fine to use the fresh stocks available in the supermarkets or buy cubes or the little stockpots. We think many of them are pretty good these days.

BREAKFAST
and
BRUNCH

1

A good breakfast is important for everyone. But if you have type 2 diabetes, or you are at risk of diabetes, it is vital to stay away from breakfast foods that are heavy on sugar and fats. Lots of packaged cereals, for instance, are packed with sweet stuff and the trad fry-up is loaded with fat. We do love our eggs, but nowadays we might opt for an omelette or an Italian-style frittata with loads of tasty veg. Avocado on toast is another favourite of ours, and if we do eat granola we make our own. That way we can make sure it's not full of sugar. If you're short of time, how about making one of our special smoothies? Just whizz it up and go. All these recipes will keep you satisfied until lunchtime without breaking the calorie bank.

Stove-top granola 16

Smoothies 18

Avocado on toast 22

Vegetable frittata 24

Smoked haddock omelette 26

Mediterranean biker brunch 28

Quick Mexican eggs 30

Buckwheat pancakes with eggs
and mushrooms 32

Corned beef hash 36

STOVE-TOP GRANOLA

When we first started dieting it was a real shock to find out that what we thought was a healthy granola breakfast actually had twice the calories of a fry-up! The best idea is to make your own granola, so you can keep the sugar down. This version is cooked in a frying pan and takes minutes to put together. We think jumbo oats work best, as they give a chunkier texture. (*See photo on colour plate A.*)

213 calories per serving (without milk or yoghurt)
Serves 6

---

1 tbsp maple syrup
20g butter
150g jumbo oats
pinch of salt
1 tbsp sunflower seeds
2 tbsp flaked almonds
50g dried fruit

Put the maple syrup and butter in a large, preferably non-stick, frying pan and melt them together over a low heat.

Add the jumbo oats with a pinch of salt. Stir until the oats are completely coated with the melted syrup and butter, then turn up the heat to medium. Spread the oats evenly over the base of the pan, leave them for about 20 seconds, then stir and repeat. Keep doing this until all the oats have turned a golden brown and smell nutty – this will take about 5 minutes.

Add the sunflower seeds, nuts and dried fruit and stir for a couple of minutes longer. Tip the granola on to a plate and let it cool for 5 minutes. The oats will crisp up more.

Serve at once with milk or yoghurt and store any leftovers in an airtight container for another time.

SMOOTHIES

You can't say us Bikers don't move with the times – we're well up with smoothies. These make a proper get-up-and-go breakfast and you can take them to work with you if you like. (*See photo on colour plate B.*)

Apple and oat smoothie

275 calories per serving
Serves 2

---

2 eating apples, cored and roughly chopped
squeeze of lemon juice
2 tbsp porridge oats
200ml fat-free yoghurt
300ml semi-skimmed milk
½ tsp cinnamon
1 tsp honey

Put the chopped apples in a blender and add a squeeze of lemon juice. Add all the remaining ingredients and blitz until the mixture is as smooth as you can get it. Divide between 2 glasses and serve at once.

Green smoothie

70 calories per serving

Serves 2

50g spinach

1 celery stick, roughly chopped

1 apple, roughly chopped

juice of 1 orange

juice of 1 lime

½ tsp grated fresh root ginger

handful of ice cubes

Wash the spinach and put it in a blender with the rest of the ingredients. Blitz until smooth, then divide between 2 glasses and serve at once.

Banana, strawberry and blueberry smoothie

103 calories per serving

Serves 2

---

1 banana, peeled

100g strawberries, hulled

100g blueberries

50ml low-fat natural yoghurt

handful of ice cubes

Put all the ingredients in a blender. Blitz until smooth, then divide between 2 glasses and serve at once.

It's so easy to make your own smoothies. Some of the ready-made versions are expensive and can be full of sugar, so high in calories.

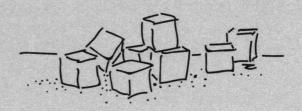

AVOCADO ON TOAST

Avo on toast is not just for trendy types. We've been enjoying it for years – sometimes with a poached egg on top for a really satisfying breakfast. In this recipe, the avocado is poshed up with some extra flavours to make it super special. Za'atar is a beautifully fragrant Middle Eastern spice. It's available in lots of supermarkets now, but if you don't have any or can't find it, it's fine to leave it out. (*See photo on colour plate B.*)

272 calories per serving
Serves 4

---

4 slices of wholemeal bread
2 avocados
juice of ½ lemon
16 cherry tomatoes, quartered
1 tsp grated lemon zest
1 tsp olive oil
a few dashes of mild vinegar (brown rice vinegar is good)
a few dashes of hot sauce
small bunch of coriander or parsley
pinches of smoked paprika
pinches of za'atar (optional)
½ tsp sesame seeds
freshly ground black pepper

Toast the bread. Roughly mash the avocados in a bowl with the lemon juice and spread the mixture over the slices of toast.

Toss the cherry tomatoes with the lemon zest, olive oil, vinegar and hot sauce. Tear the coriander or parsley leaves and mix them with the tomatoes. Season with black pepper, then divide them between the avocado-covered toast.

Sprinkle with pinches of paprika, za'atar, if using, and sesame seeds and serve immediately.

VEGETABLE FRITTATA

A frittata is simply the Italian version of an omelette. It's finished off under the grill and it's mega good. We like to roast most of the veg for extra flavour and you can cook them the night before if you want a quick brunch dish for the morning. Vary the veg as you fancy – asparagus, peas and mushrooms are all good – but stay way from the spuds and keep your calorie count in mind.

230 calories per serving
Serves 4

---

2 red onions, cut into wedges

1 courgette, cut into rounds

1 red pepper, deseeded and cut into strips

200g butternut squash, peeled and diced

1 tbsp olive oil

1 tsp dried oregano

½ head of broccoli, broken into small florets

50g green beans, cut in half

6 eggs, beaten

low-cal olive oil spray

6 cherry tomatoes, halved

handful of fresh basil leaves, torn

freshly ground black pepper

First roast the veg. Preheat the oven to 200°C/Fan 180°C/Gas 6. Line a baking tray or roasting dish with non-stick baking paper and spread the onions, courgette, red pepper and butternut squash over it. Drizzle over the olive oil, then turn the vegetables over with your hands, making sure they are all lightly coated with oil. Sprinkle with the oregano. Place the baking tray in the oven and roast the vegetables for 30 minutes, then set aside.

Bring a small pan of water to the boil and blanch the broccoli and beans for 2 minutes, then drain. Season the eggs with black pepper.

Heat your grill to its highest setting. Lightly spray a large non-stick frying pan with oil and place the pan over a medium heat. Tip the roasted veg into the frying pan and spread them out as evenly as you can, so that each quarter gets a good balance of the different vegetables. Add the broccoli, green beans and cherry tomatoes and sprinkle over the torn basil.

Pour the eggs over the vegetables. Cook over a medium heat until the base of the frittata has set – you'll see the edges starting to turn brown. Place the pan under the hot grill and cook for a few more minutes until the eggs have set and the top of the frittata has started to puff up slightly. Remove the pan carefully – the handle will be hot – cut the frittata into quarters and serve. It's good cold too.

SMOKED HADDOCK OMELETTE

The idea for this recipe came from a dish known as omelette Arnold Bennett, after the famous novelist. It was created for him by the Savoy Hotel in London and became a much-loved classic. Our version is much less calorific than the original but is still very good to eat and packed with protein for a sustaining meal. Great for brunch – or any time of day.

428 calories per serving (2)
285 calories per serving (3)
Serves 2–3

200g smoked haddock fillet (preferably undyed)

250ml semi-skimmed milk

1 tbsp cornflour

1 tbsp reduced-fat crème fraiche

1 tbsp finely chopped chives

low-cal olive oil spray

5 eggs, beaten

25g reduced-fat Cheddar cheese, grated

freshly ground black pepper

Put the haddock in a wide pan and pour in the milk to cover. Bring to the boil, cover, then turn off the heat and leave to stand for 10 minutes. Strain the milk into a jug. When the fish is cool enough to handle, break it up into chunks and set it aside. Discard the skin and any stray bones.

Mix the cornflour with a little cold water until you have a smooth paste. Measure 150ml of the cooking milk into a small saucepan and add the crème fraiche. Pour in the cornflour mixture and stir over a gentle heat until you have a thick sauce. Season with pepper, then stir in the haddock and the chopped chives.

Heat a large frying pan and spray it lightly with oil. Pour in the beaten eggs, making sure the whole of the base of the frying pan is evenly covered. When the egg mixture is almost set, pile the haddock mixture over one half of the omelette and sprinkle the cheese on top. Carefully flip the uncovered half of the omelette over the filling and leave to cook for a couple of minutes until the cheese has melted. Cut the omelette in half or divide into thirds and serve at once.

MEDITERRANEAN BIKER BRUNCH

This is our version of a dish called piperade from the Basque region in the Pyrenees. We've fiddled about a bit, added some fennel and other extra flavours and come up with what we think is a real winner, with plenty of veg to boost your five a day. You can make the veg in advance if you like, then reheat them and add the eggs. (*See photo on colour plate A.*)

153 calories per serving
Serves 4

10ml olive oil

1 red and 1 green pepper, deseeded and cut into strips

1 fennel bulb, trimmed and cut into thin wedges

1 tsp fennel seeds

½ tsp coriander seeds

½ tsp chilli flakes

1 piece of thinly pared orange zest

400g can of tomatoes, or fresh equivalent

4 eggs

1 tsp white wine vinegar

a few basil leaves, torn, to serve

freshly ground black pepper

Heat the oil in a large frying pan with a lid. Add the peppers and fennel wedges with a splash of water, cover the pan and cook for 10–15 minutes, stirring regularly.

Lightly crush the fennel seeds and coriander seeds. Add them to the pan with the chilli flakes, orange zest and plenty of pepper, then add the tomatoes and stir. Add another splash of water and simmer gently until the peppers and fennel are tender and the sauce is nicely reduced.

To poach the eggs, half fill a saucepan with water, and add the wine vinegar. Bring the water to the boil, then carefully lower the eggs (still in their shells) into the water and leave them for exactly 20 seconds. Remove the eggs from the water.

Turn the heat down so the water is barely simmering. Carefully crack each egg into the water and cook them for 3 minutes. Once the eggs are cooked they will rise to the surface. Remove the eggs from the pan and put them on some kitchen paper to drain before serving.

Remove the piece of orange zest, then serve the veg topped with the eggs and basil leaves.

QUICK MEXICAN EGGS

This Mexican feast – known as huevos rancheros or ranchers' eggs – is one of our very favourite dishes for breakfast, brunch or any time of day really! Proper refried beans take a while but our super-quick version is ready in minutes.

356 calories per serving
Serves 4

BEANS
1 tsp olive oil
1 garlic clove, crushed
1 tsp oregano
1 tsp ground cumin
1 tbsp tomato purée
400g can of black beans, drained but not rinsed
freshly ground black pepper

SALSA
juice of 1 lime
1 avocado, flesh diced

To serve
4 corn tortillas
low-cal olive oil spray

4 eggs
½ tsp smoked chilli powder
small bunch of coriander, chopped

First prepare the beans. Heat the oil in a small saucepan and add the garlic. Cook for 30 seconds, then add the oregano, cumin and tomato purée. Continue to cook until the purée starts to separate, then add the beans along with 100ml of water. Season the beans with pepper and leave them to simmer gently while you get everything else ready.

For the salsa, put the lime juice in a bowl, add the avocado and stir to combine.

Now warm the tortillas. Sprinkle each tortilla with water and place it in a dry frying pan for 10–15 seconds, then flip and repeat. Wrap the tortillas in a tea towel to keep them warm. Spritz a frying pan with oil. Add the eggs and fry them gently until they are cooked as you like them. Sprinkle each one with a little chilli powder.

Divide the beans between 4 plates and top with the eggs. Serve with the tortillas and salsa and garnish with plenty of chopped coriander. That's it!

BIKER TIP _____
If you like, add a bag of baby spinach leaves to the beans, stirring them through until the leaves wilt.

BUCKWHEAT PANCAKES WITH EGGS AND MUSHROOMS

Buckwheat flour makes great pancakes – known as galettes to our friends in Brittany – and it's available in supermarkets. Despite the name, it's not actually a wheat and it's gluten-free, so it's good for those with wheat allergies. The batter makes eight pancakes, but it freezes well or can be kept in the fridge for a few days. (*See photo on colour plate A.*)

75 calories per pancake
193 calories with filling
Serves 4

PANCAKES

100g buckwheat flour
pinch of salt
1 large egg
300ml semi-skimmed milk
low-cal olive oil spray

FILLING

1 tbsp olive oil
100g mushrooms, wiped clean and thinly sliced

1 garlic clove, finely chopped
1 tbsp finely chopped fresh parsley
4 eggs
freshly ground black pepper

To make the batter, sift the flour into a bowl and stir in the salt. Make a well in the flour and break in the egg, then gradually incorporate the flour into the egg until you have a thick paste.

Start mixing in the milk, little by little, until you have a smooth batter. If you have time, leave the batter to stand for about an hour, but don't worry if you can't.

To make the filling, heat the oil in a non-stick frying pan and add the mushrooms. Fry until they are tender, then add the garlic and parsley. Season with pepper and cook for another minute or so, then tip everything into a bowl. Set the pan aside for cooking the eggs later.

To make the pancakes, heat a small non-stick frying pan over a medium heat and spritz lightly with oil. Hold the pan in one hand and add a small ladleful of batter (about 2 tablespoons), swirling quickly so the entire base of the pan is coated. Cook the pancake on one side until lots of little air bubbles appear and a palette knife slides easily under it.

CONTINUED ON NEXT PAGE

Flip the pancake over and cook on the other side for about half a minute, then slide on to a plate. Make 3 more pancakes in the same way. You shouldn't need to add more oil to the pan – the remaining pancakes will brown more quickly, but just turn down the heat a little and keep a close eye on them.

Break the eggs into the pan you used to cook the mushrooms and fry them gently until the whites are set and the yolks are still runny.

Put one of the pancakes back into the pancake pan. Put a quarter of the mushrooms in the centre and top with an egg. Turn the edges of the pancake into the centre – they won't meet so you'll see the filling peeking through the gap. Transfer to a warm plate. Fill the rest of the pancakes in the same way and serve immediately.

Pour any batter you don't use into an airtight plastic container and freeze for another time.

We love mushrooms. They're low in calories, but satisfying, and even the ordinary white button kind contain lots of vitamins and minerals.

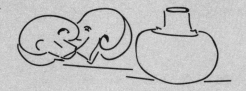

CORNED BEEF HASH

This is a proper feast of a breakfast and by using carrot and celeriac instead of potato, you cut down the calories and add extra flavour. We usually make this with a can of corned beef, which is great stuff, but we've also tried it with leftover home-made corned beef and it's even better. There's a recipe in our *Meat Feasts* book if you want to try it. It's not as fatty as the canned beef either. (*See photo on colour plate B.*)

248 calories per serving
Serves 4

200g celeriac, finely diced

200g carrots, finely diced

1 tsp vegetable oil

1 onion, finely chopped

200g can of lean or reduced-fat corned beef
   or equivalent, diced

1 tbsp tomato purée

1 tsp Dijon mustard

100ml beef stock

1 tsp Worcestershire sauce

low-cal olive oil spray

4 eggs

Put the celeriac and carrots in a saucepan and pour over just-boiled water to cover. Bring the water back to the boil, cover the pan and cook the vegetables for 7 minutes. They should be just cooked through. Drain thoroughly.

Meanwhile, heat the oil in a large frying pan. Add the onion and cook it over a medium heat until it starts to soften. As soon as the vegetables are ready, add them to the frying pan along with the corned beef. Cook for 5 minutes until a crust has formed on the bottom of the mixture.

Put the tomato purée and mustard into a small bowl or jug with the beef stock and Worcestershire sauce and whisk well. Pour this mixture over the corned beef and vegetables and stir thoroughly. Cook for another 10 minutes, stirring every so often, until there are plenty of crusty brown bits interspersed through the mix.

While the hash finishes cooking, heat another frying pan and spritz it with oil. Add the eggs and fry them until the whites have just set. Serve the hash with the eggs on top.

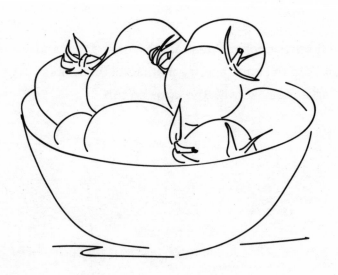

SOUPS
and
SALADS

2

A good bowl of warming, comforting soup or a big plateful of crunchy salad are both perfect for lunchtime – or at any time of day. There's something about soup that helps you feel fuller for longer, and all our soup recipes are low in calories but high in flavour – ideal if you want to lose weight. Our salads are super-tasty and sustaining, as most contain some grains, pulses or protein, and they are a great way of upping your veg intake – really important if you are suffering from diabetes. They're perfect for lunch on the go too. Make a big batch of soup at the start of the week and take some to work, along with a box of salad. You'll keep the hunger pangs at bay and feel ready for anything.

Tomato soup 42

Pea, lettuce and asparagus soup 44

Courgette, mint and lemon soup 46

Red lentil and harissa soup 48

Bean and vegetable soup 50

Chunky chicken soup 54

Scotch broth 56

Roasted carrot, pepper and chickpea salad 58

Summery green coleslaw 60

Tabbouleh 62

Harissa vegetables and jumbo couscous 64

Smoked trout salad 68

Chicken, squash and quinoa salad 70

TOMATO SOUP

Our tomato soup is really rich and creamy but there's no cream in it and no sugar – just lots of veg and lots of flavour. The fennel seeds add an extra tasty tang but if you don't have any, or don't like them, just leave them out. You could also chill this soup and keep it in the fridge to enjoy cold as a snack. (*See photo on colour plate C.*)

171 calories per serving
Serves 4

---

1 tbsp olive oil
1 onion, diced
1 celery stick, trimmed and diced
1 large carrot, diced
1 leek, trimmed and thinly sliced
100g butternut squash, diced
200g celeriac, diced
1 tsp fennel seeds, ground (optional)
2 garlic cloves, finely chopped
50g red lentils
1.2 litres vegetable or chicken stock
400g can of tomatoes
handful of basil leaves, torn
freshly ground black pepper

Heat the oil in a large pan and add the onion, celery, carrot, leek, squash and celeriac. Cook gently over a fairly high heat, stirring regularly, until the vegetables start to brown slightly around the edges and give off a sweet aroma.

Add the fennel seeds, if using, and the garlic and cook for another 2 minutes. Add the red lentils and pour over the stock, then season with pepper. Simmer for 10 minutes.

Add the tomatoes and simmer for another 10–15 minutes until the lentils are completely soft. Add the basil leaves and let them wilt into the soup, then remove the pan from the heat. Purée the soup until smooth, adding more stock or water if it seems too thick for your liking. Check for seasoning before serving and add a little more pepper to taste.

BIKER TIP

This soup is ideal for freezing in individual portions, ready to defrost for a super-quick lunch.

PEA, LETTUCE AND ASPARAGUS SOUP

Get your fill of chlorophyll – this soup makes you feel healthy just by looking at it! It's an ideal quick, low-calorie meal and the short cooking time keeps the colour fresh and green. (*See photo on colour plate D.*)

220 calories per serving
Serves 4

---

1 tbsp olive oil

1 leek, trimmed and finely diced

100g thin asparagus spears

2 little gem lettuces, shredded

600g frozen peas or petits pois

1 litre hot vegetable stock

squeeze of lemon or lime juice

freshly ground black pepper

HERB CREAM

2 tbsp single cream

small bunch of basil or mint

Heat the oil in a large saucepan. Add the diced leek and a splash of water, then put a lid on the pan and cook over a low heat for 5 minutes.

Cut the tips off the asparagus and set them aside for later. Finely slice the remaining stems and add these to the leeks, along with the shredded lettuce. Cook for another couple of minutes, then add the peas and pour the hot stock into the pan. Season with black pepper and leave the soup to simmer for 5 minutes.

While the soup is simmering, heat a griddle until it's very hot and grill the asparagus tips until they're nicely charred.

Blend the soup to a smooth texture. Taste, then add a little lemon or lime juice – just enough to bring out the flavour.

If you have a mini blender or food processor, blitz the cream with the basil or mint, but if not, just finely chop the herbs and stir them into the cream. Serve the soup drizzled with a little of the herb cream and topped with the grilled asparagus tips.

COURGETTE, MINT AND LEMON SOUP

Courgette soups are often made with milk or cream and are quite rich, but we've kept ours nice and fresh and simple. If you're a vegan, this is one for you and if not, try it anyway as it's really tasty, super-green and keeps you lean. (*See photo on colour plate C.*)

105 calories per serving
Serves 6

---

1 tbsp olive oil

1 onion, finely chopped

1 potato, finely diced

750g courgettes, coarsely grated

2 garlic cloves, finely chopped

grated zest of 1 lemon

1 tsp dried mint

750ml vegetable stock

100g frozen peas

100g baby spinach

squeeze of lemon juice (optional)

freshly ground black pepper

Heat the olive oil in a large saucepan, add the onion and potato and stir well to coat them in the oil. Add a splash of water, cover the pan and cook the veg gently for about 10 minutes. Add the courgettes, garlic, lemon zest and mint, then cook for another 2 minutes.

Pour in the stock, season with black pepper and bring to the boil. Simmer for about 5 minutes, then add the peas and spinach. Cook for another 2 minutes until the spinach has completely wilted and the peas are just tender but still a lovely fresh green colour.

Purée the soup in a blender or with a stick blender, but be careful not to over process it, as you want to keep some flecks of green throughout. Taste and add a squeeze of lemon juice, if using, and more pepper if you like before serving.

If you want to make your soup a bit more fancy, decorate it with ribbons of courgette and some extra lemon zest.

RED LENTIL AND HARISSA SOUP

Quick to prepare, this soup packs a punch of flavour and warms the cockles on a cold day. The nice little seasoning of lemon, garlic and coriander adds a bit of oomph to the soup. (*See photo on colour plate C.*)

166 calories per serving
Serves 6

---

1 tbsp olive oil

1 large onion, finely chopped

2 garlic cloves, finely chopped

2 tbsp finely chopped coriander stems

1–2 tbsp harissa paste (depending on how much heat
   you want)

200g red lentils, rinsed

1 litre vegetable stock

400g can of tomatoes

squeeze of lemon (optional)

freshly ground black pepper

HERBY DRESSING

zest of 1 lemon
1 garlic clove, finely chopped
coriander leaves, finely chopped

Heat the oil in a large pan. Add the onion and cook it over a gentle heat until softened. Add the garlic and cook for another minute, then stir in the coriander stems and the harissa paste.

Add the lentils and stir until they are coated with the paste, then pour over the stock and season with pepper.

Bring the stock to the boil, then turn the heat down and simmer for about 10 minutes. Add the tomatoes and simmer for another 10 minutes. Stir and check the consistency of the soup – add a splash more water if it seems too thick. Taste and add more pepper and a squeeze of lemon juice if you think the soup needs it.

To make the herby dressing, finely chop the lemon zest, garlic and coriander together until well combined.

Blend the soup if you want it smooth – the lentils will have broken down enough to thicken it, but there will still be some texture from the onions and tomatoes. Serve with the dressing spooned over the top.

BEAN AND VEGETABLE SOUP

Our version of ribollita, a classic Italian recipe, this is a good hearty soup that'll keep you going for hours. We've used less pasta than in the traditional recipe to keep the calories down, but there are plenty of beans and vegetables to fill you up. Use any sort of cabbage you like, including spring greens, kale or Swiss chard, but don't be tempted to try spinach, as it will just end up as mush. This is also a great recipe for using up a Parmesan rind if you have one in the fridge. It doesn't matter how hard and dried up it is, it will still bring a nice bit of extra flavour to your soup. (*See photo on colour plate D.*)

290 calories per serving
Serves 4

---

1 tbsp olive oil

50g back bacon, trimmed of fat and finely diced

1 onion, finely chopped

1 fennel bulb, trimmed and finely chopped

2 carrots, finely chopped

2 celery sticks, chopped

4 garlic cloves, finely chopped

1 tsp dried oregano

Parmesan rind (optional)

100ml red wine

400g can of cannellini beans, drained and rinsed

4 fresh tomatoes, finely chopped, or 200g canned chopped
   tomatoes

600ml chicken stock

50g wholewheat pasta (any short form will do)

½ green cabbage or the equivalent in other greens

1 large courgette, diagonally sliced

squeeze of lemon juice (optional)

freshly ground black pepper

To serve

handful of basil leaves, torn

25g Parmesan cheese, grated

Heat the oil in a large saucepan. Add the diced bacon and fry
until it is nice and crisp and brown. Then add the onion, fennel,
carrots, celery and garlic to the pan and cook gently for a
couple of minutes.

Sprinkle over the oregano, add the Parmesan rind, if using,
then pour over the red wine. Bring to the boil and simmer
until the wine has reduced by about half.

CONTINUED ON NEXT PAGE

Add the beans and tomatoes, then pour in the stock. Bring the soup back to the boil and simmer for about 15 minutes until all the vegetables are tender.

Add the pasta and cabbage, continue to simmer for 5 minutes, then add the courgette. Simmer for another 5–10 minutes until the pasta is cooked but still has a little bite to it and all the vegetables are cooked through. Have a taste and add more black pepper and a squeeze of lemon juice if you think the soup needs it.

Sprinkle over the basil and serve the soup with a scant tablespoon of grated Parmesan on each bowlful.

Not all your veg has to be fresh. Frozen vegetables are fine, as are time savers like canned tomatoes.

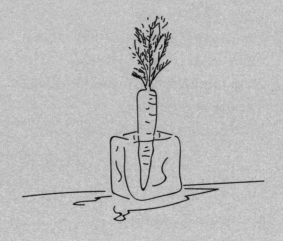

CHUNKY CHICKEN SOUP

If you've got some leftover roast chicken in your fridge this is a great way to use it. This soup is so nourishing and the spices and ginger give it a lovely warming flavour. It feels good for you and it tastes epic.

306 calories per serving

Serves 4

---

2 tsp olive oil

2 red onions, cut into wedges

2 large carrots, cut into chunks

40g basmati rice, rinsed

3 garlic cloves, finely chopped

30g chunk of fresh root ginger, finely chopped

¼ tsp turmeric

¼ tsp cinnamon

1 litre chicken stock

1 large sweet potato, cut into chunks

200g chard or kale, shredded

200g roast chicken, pulled into chunks

squeeze of lemon juice

freshly ground black pepper

Heat the oil in a large pan and add the onions and carrots. Cook them gently over a high heat for a few minutes until they're starting to take on some colour, then add the rice, garlic, ginger and spices. Stir to combine, add the chicken stock and season with black pepper.

Bring the soup to the boil, then turn the heat down to a simmer and cook until the vegetables and rice are al dente – this will take 10–12 minutes.

Add the sweet potato, greens and chicken. Cover the pan and leave the soup to cook for another 10 minutes until the sweet potato and greens are tender. Taste for seasoning and add the lemon juice before serving.

BIKER TIP

If you don't have any leftover roast chicken, you could make this soup with some cooked chicken from the supermarket.

SCOTCH BROTH

Some recipes for this gutsy, nourishing Scottish classic use just lamb stock, while others include meat from neck fillet or other cuts. Neck is fatty so we use diced lamb leg meat to add flavour and texture to the soup, along with loads of luscious veg and barley. We think it's best to soak the peas overnight, then boil them for ten minutes before adding them to the soup to be on the safe side. You don't want to end up with tough little green bullets in your soup! (*See photo on colour plate D.*)

240 calories per serving
Serves 6

50g split green peas, soaked overnight

400g lean lamb leg meat, finely diced

1.2 litres lamb stock or water

50g pearl barley

4 carrots, finely diced

2 onions, finely diced

2 celery sticks, trimmed and finely diced

½ swede, finely diced

1 large turnip, finely diced

1 thyme sprig

1 bay leaf

½ cabbage, shredded (white, green or savoy)

2 leeks, halved lengthways and finely sliced
freshly ground black pepper

Soak the split green peas overnight in plenty of water. When you are ready to start making the Scotch broth, drain the peas and put them in a saucepan. Cover with cold water, bring to the boil and boil hard for 10 minutes, then drain and set aside. The peas are now ready to use.

Put the lamb in a large pan or flameproof casserole dish, cover it with the stock and bring everything to the boil. Skim off any brown foam that collects on the surface and keep doing this until the foam turns white. Add the pearl barley, boiled split peas, carrots, onions, celery, swede, turnip and herbs, then season with pepper and bring back to the boil. Turn the heat down to a low simmer and cook gently for an hour, adding more liquid if necessary.

Add the cabbage and leeks to the pan and simmer for another 15 minutes until they are just tender. Serve the Scotch broth in deep bowls.

ROASTED CARROT, PEPPER AND CHICKPEA SALAD

This salad and its zingy citrusy dressing are great served with some plain grilled meat, but we also love it on its own for a yummy light lunch. A green salad alongside is good. (*See photo on colour plate E.*)

136 calories per serving
Serves 4

---

2 large carrots, cut into 2cm chunks

1 tsp ground cumin

1 tsp olive oil

2 red peppers, seeded and cut in half, lengthways

400g can of chickpeas, drained and rinsed

2 tbsp chopped dill

2 tbsp chopped mint

2 tbsp chopped parsley or coriander

freshly ground black pepper

DRESSING

1 tsp tahini

1 tsp olive oil

freshly squeezed juice of 1 orange

1 garlic clove, crushed

¼ tsp allspice

½ tsp cumin

Preheat the oven to 220°C/Fan 200°C/Gas 7. Line a roasting dish with baking paper.

Bring a pan of water to the boil, add the carrots and simmer for 15 minutes until they're almost tender. Drain the carrots and tip them into the roasting dish, then season with pepper and cumin. Drizzle with the olive oil.

Push the carrots into one half of the roasting dish and put the peppers in the other half, cut-side down. Roast for 20 minutes until the carrots have taken on some colour and the peppers are starting to soften and look slightly charred. Remove the dish from the oven and put the peppers in a bowl, cover and leave them to steam until they are cool enough to handle. Peel off the skin – it should come off easily – and cut or tear the peppers into thin strips.

To make the dressing, whisk all the ingredients together and season with pepper

To assemble the salad, put the carrots, peppers and chickpeas in a large bowl. Add all the herbs, then pour over the dressing. Gently mix everything together, then leave the salad to stand at room temperature for a while to allow the flavours develop before serving.

SUMMERY GREEN COLESLAW

Fresh, crunchy and full of flavour, this green coleslaw really smacks of summer. It's really nice with lots of herbs but it's best to add them just before serving, as they will start to go black and limp after being torn and chopped. (*See photo on colour plate E.*)

130 calories per serving
Serves 4

100g frozen peas or baby broad beans
1 small green cabbage, shredded
1 large courgette, grated or sliced into matchsticks
1 large fennel bulb, trimmed and sliced into matchsticks
1 bunch of spring onions, finely sliced
2 celery sticks, finely chopped
1 green apple, grated
juice of ½ lime
freshly ground black pepper

To serve
handful bunch of basil leaves, torn
bunch of mint leaves, chopped

DRESSING

2 tbsp low-fat yoghurt

2 tbsp reduced-fat mayonnaise

zest and juice of 1 lemon

1 tbsp finely chopped tarragon

Bring a pan of water to the boil, add the peas or broad beans and bring the water back to the boil. Cook them for 2 minutes, then drain.

Put the cabbage, courgette, fennel, spring onions and celery in a large bowl and add the cooked peas or beans. Mix the grated apple with the lime juice, then add it to the vegetables. Season with pepper, then stir well to combine.

Whisk together all the dressing ingredients and season with pepper. Pour the dressing over the vegetables. Garnish with the basil and mint leaves just before serving.

TABBOULEH

An authentic tabbouleh contains very little bulgur wheat but lots and lots of fresh herbs, and ours is no exception. This is great on its own, with a group of other salad dishes or with some simple grilled chicken. The celeriac adds extra texture, but if you don't like it – or can't get hold of any – just use an extra courgette.

101 calories per serving (4)
68 calories per serving (6)
Serves 4–6

---

1 red onion, finely chopped

30g bulgur wheat

100g celeriac, peeled

2 courgettes

200g large, ripe red tomatoes, finely chopped

1 red pepper, deseeded and finely diced

large bunch of flatleaf parsley, finely sliced (not chopped)

small bunch of mint, leaves only, finely sliced

DRESSING

1 tbsp olive oil

juice of 1 lemon

pinch of cinnamon

1 tsp ground cumin

freshly ground black pepper

Put the finely chopped red onion in a bowl and cover with cold water, then leave to stand for 20 minutes. This takes the harshness out of the onions and makes the flavour more mellow. Soak the bulgur wheat in a bowl of just-boiled water for 5 minutes, then drain and set aside.

Cut the celeriac into chunks. Top and tail the courgettes and cut them into chunks too. Put the celeriac in a food processor and pulse a few times, then add the courgettes and pulse again until everything is the size of large breadcrumbs.

Drain the onion and put it in a bowl with the celeriac, courgettes, tomatoes and pepper, then stir in the herbs. Whisk all the dressing ingredients together and pour over the vegetables. Stir, then leave to stand for a few minutes before eating. This salad is best served at room temperature.

HARISSA VEGETABLES AND JUMBO COUSCOUS

Spicy harissa paste adds a lovely punch of flavour to these vegetables and the two dishes make a perfect combo. Jumbo couscous was new to us but it's a wonderful thing – you don't need a lot to give a salad lots of body and texture. It's great with these vegetables but you can also enjoy it by itself for lunch or with some grilled fish for supper. (*See photo on colour plate E.*)

197 calories per serving
Serves 4

---

1 tsp olive oil

2 red onions, finely sliced into wedges

2 red peppers, deseeded and cut into strips

2 large courgettes, thinly sliced on the diagonal

zest of 1 lemon

1 tsp cumin seeds

1 tbsp tomato purée

1 tbsp harissa paste

100ml hot vegetable stock or water

12 cherry tomatoes, halved

COUSCOUS AND SALAD
500ml vegetable stock
100g wholewheat jumbo couscous
200g salad leaves
squeeze of lemon juice
handful of mint leaves
handful of parsley leaves
freshly ground black pepper

Heat the oil in a large frying pan. Add the onions and red peppers and fry them over a high heat for 5 minutes. Add the courgettes, then continue to cook for another couple of minutes.

Add the lemon zest and cumin seeds. Whisk the tomato purée with the harissa paste and the 100ml of stock or water, then pour this over the vegetables and cover the pan. Turn the heat down and simmer for another 5 minutes until the vegetables are softened but still with a bit of bite to them.

While the vegetables are cooking, pour the 500ml of hot vegetable stock or water into a pan, add the couscous and season it with pepper. Bring it to the boil, cover the pan and simmer for 6–8 minutes until the couscous has plumped up and is tender. Remove the pan from the heat and drain off any remaining liquid.

CONTINUED ON NEXT PAGE

Add the tomatoes to the frying pan with the vegetables and leave them to soften, covered, for a further minute.

Mix the couscous with the salad leaves, then add the vegetables and their dressing. Squeeze over a little lemon juice and sprinkle liberally with the mint and parsley leaves.

BIKER TIP

If you like, you can make this salad even lower in calories by replacing the couscous with cauliflower. Divide the cauli into florets and put them in a food processor. Blitz to the texture of fine breadcrumbs.

Try to include a wide range of vegetables in your meals to make sure you get a good balance of vitamins and minerals.

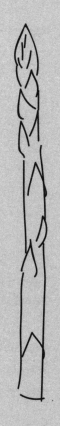

SMOKED TROUT SALAD

Fillets of smoked trout make a quick, easy and nourishing salad and the celeriac fries add a crispy crunch. Get those going right away so they can be cooking while you prepare the rest of the salad and you'll be sitting down to a tasty feast in no time. You need hot-smoked trout (or salmon) for this, as it flakes nicely. Thinly sliced fish doesn't work.

135 calories per serving
Serves 4

200g celeriac, peeled

low-cal olive oil spray

100g green beans

100g salad leaves, such as spinach, baby kale, pea shoots or lamb's lettuce

250g cooked beetroot, cut into wedges

200g smoked trout

small bunch of dill, leaves only

a few chives

freshly ground black pepper

DRESSING

75ml buttermilk or low-fat yoghurt

1 tsp cider vinegar

2 tsp Dijon mustard

pinch of sugar-free sweetener (optional)

Preheat the oven to 220°C/Fan 200°C/Gas 7. Cut the celeriac into very fine matchsticks. The easiest way to do this is to cut it into thin slices first, using a mandolin if you have one, and then into fine strips. Spritz a baking tray with low-cal oil and spread the celeriac strips over it. Sprinkle them quite generously with pepper, then spritz with oil again.

Bake the celeriac fries in the oven for 20 minutes, turning them over every 5 minutes or so, until they have shrunk down and cooked through. You will find some strips are well browned and crunchy while others are slightly softer, but the contrast is good. The fries will crisp up further as they cool.

While the celeriac is cooking, prepare the rest of the salad. Trim the green beans and cut them in half. Cook them in a saucepan of boiling water for 4–5 minutes or until tender, then drain.

Spread the salad leaves over a large platter and add the beans, beetroot and celeriac fries.

Break up the trout into chunks and add these to the salad. Separate the dill into small fronds and snip the chives with scissors, then sprinkle them over the salad.

Whisk the salad dressing ingredients together and season with pepper. Drizzle the dressing over the salad and serve.

CHICKEN, SQUASH AND QUINOA SALAD

You can buy cooked quinoa or we like to cook up a big batch and keep some in the freezer – it's always good to have some handy for a hearty salad like this one. Then all you have to do is roast the squash and put everything together. Lunch sorted!

295 calories per serving
Serves 4

300g butternut squash, diced

1 tsp olive oil

½ tsp dried oregano

½ garlic bulb, cloves separated but unpeeled

150g cooked quinoa

200g baby salad leaves

200g cooked chicken, diced

1 avocado, peeled and diced

bunch of spring onions, sliced into rounds

handful of mint leaves, to serve

freshly ground black pepper

DRESSING

2 tsp olive oil

zest and juice of 1 lime

1 tsp red wine vinegar

pinch of sugar-free sweetener (optional)

½ tsp chipotle powder (or other chilli powder)

Preheat the oven to 200°C/Fan 180°C/Gas 6. Put the squash in a roasting tin and drizzle it with the olive oil. Season well with pepper, sprinkle over the oregano and add the garlic cloves. Roast the squash for about 25 minutes, until it's just tender and slightly browned around the edge. Remove the garlic and set the squash aside to cool to room temperature.

Now make the dressing. Squash the garlic flesh out of the roasted cloves and put it all in a bowl. Add the remaining dressing ingredients, season with pepper, then whisk everything together.

Arrange the quinoa and salad leaves on a large platter and add the chicken, avocado, spring onions and roasted squash. Drizzle over the salad dressing, then top with the mint leaves. Serve at once.

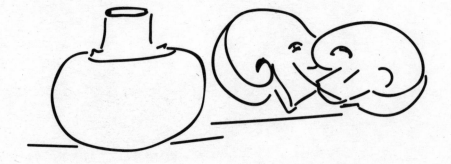

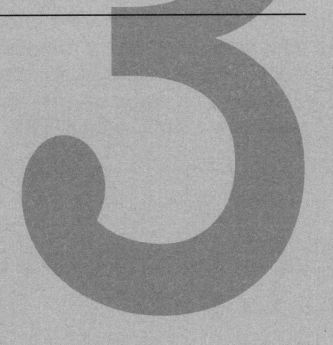

SNACKS
and
DIPS

Snacking used to be our downfall. We found that the danger was that if we got too hungry and didn't have anything healthy to hand, we were all too easily tempted to grab a chocolate bar or a sugary biscuit, just to stop those pangs. If you do have diabetes, snacks are important for keeping your blood sugar under control, but they should be nutritious and not high in fat or sugar. Have a go at making some of these dips to keep in the fridge and enjoy them with some sticks of carrot, cucumber and red pepper. Or try some home-made popcorn or roast chickpeas. Both are full of healthy fibre and by making your own you know exactly what's in them.

Lunch-box pot noodles 76

Carrot, red pepper and butter bean dip 78

Smoked trout dip or filling 80

Tuna and caper dip or filling 82

Artichoke and lemon dip 84

Lil's roast vegetable dip 86

Socca and salsa 88

Roast chickpeas 90

Spiced popcorn 92

LUNCH-BOX POT NOODLES

Take this to the office for your lunch and your workmates will look on in envy. We've suggested three different seasonings and you'll probably come up with your own variations too – let us know! It's really important to use the right kind of noodles – you want the sort that will cook in two or three minutes. Vary your veggies as you like, but choose things that cook in about the same time as the noodles. There's no need to defrost the peas, as they will defrost when you add the hot water.

322 calories per serving
Serves 2

---

2 small nests of quick-cook noodles
1 small carrot
1 small courgette
½ red pepper
2 spring onions
4 mushrooms
1 garlic clove, finely chopped
5g chunk of fresh root ginger, finely chopped
2 tbsp frozen peas
50g cooked chicken
small bunch of fresh coriander
freshly ground black pepper

THAI SEASONING

1 chicken stock cube, crumbled

1 tbsp Thai green curry paste

1 tbsp fish sauce

juice of 1 lime

MISO SEASONING

1 tbsp instant miso

a few thin strips of nori seaweed

1 tbsp tamari or soy sauce

Divide the noodles between 2 large, lidded, heatproof jars. Grate the carrot and cut the courgette and red pepper into thin matchsticks. Thinly slice the spring onions and the mushrooms. Layer the vegetables on top of the noodles, then sprinkle over the garlic and ginger, followed by the peas. Finely dice or shred the chicken and add this too, then top with some coriander leaves.

Add the ingredients for your choice of seasoning – Thai or miso – and a little black pepper. Seal with the lid. When you are ready to cook your pot noodles, pour over freshly boiled hot water. Leave the lid sitting on top and leave for 4–5 minutes, prodding regularly with a fork or a chopstick so the seasonings mix and dissolve into the water.

When the noodles have softened, continue to mix, then eat while still hot. Season with some extra soy, fish sauce and lime juice if you like.

CARROT, RED PEPPER AND BUTTER BEAN DIP

You could use chickpeas or any other kind of bean for this but butter beans do work particularly well. There's very little oil in the dip, which saves on calories, but the crème fraiche or yoghurt really improves the texture and gives the dip great mouth feel. Serve with some radishes and sticks of crunchy carrot, cucumber and celery.

64 calories per serving
Serves 8

---

2 large carrots, cut into rounds

1 head of garlic, cloves separated but unpeeled (2 cloves reserved)

1 large red pepper, deseeded and halved

1 tsp olive oil

400g can of butter beans, drained and rinsed

1 tsp cumin

½ tsp sweet smoked paprika

¼ tsp cayenne or chilli powder

1 tsp tahini

2 tbsp reduced-fat crème fraiche or yoghurt

squeeze of lemon juice (optional)

freshly ground black pepper

1 tsp olive oil
extra paprika and cayenne

Preheat the oven to its highest temperature. Bring a pan of
water to the boil and add the carrots and garlic – having
set aside 2 of the cloves. Simmer for 15 minutes, then drain
thoroughly and spread them over half of a roasting tin. Put the
red pepper in the other half of the tin. Drizzle over the olive oil,
then put the veg in the oven and roast for about 20 minutes,
until the carrots have started to take on colour and the red
pepper is soft.

Put the red pepper in a bowl, cover and set aside. When it is
cool enough to handle, peel off the skin. Squeeze the flesh out
of the garlic cloves and put this in a food processor with the
red pepper, carrots, butter beans, cumin, paprika, cayenne or
chilli powder and the tahini. Finely chop the reserved garlic
cloves and add those too. Season with pepper.

Purée the dip until smooth, then fold in the crème fraiche or
yoghurt. Taste for seasoning and add a squeeze of lemon juice
if you like. Scoop the dip into a bowl and serve drizzled with a
teaspoon of oil and sprinkled with a little paprika and cayenne.

SMOKED TROUT DIP OR FILLING

You'll find smoked trout fillets in every supermarket and they make a really tasty dip or sandwich or wrap filling that's really quick and easy to make. (*See photo on colour plate G.*)

58 **calories per serving (dip)**
146 **calories per open sandwich**
157 **calories per wrap**
Makes 4 servings of dip, 4 open sandwiches or 2 wraps

150g smoked trout fillets
2 tbsp reduced-fat crème fraiche
1 tsp horseradish sauce
¼ cucumber, peeled, deseeded and chopped
1 tbsp finely chopped dill
squeeze of lemon juice (optional)
freshly ground black pepper

OPEN SANDWICHES
2 cooked beetroots, thinly sliced
4 slices of wholemeal or rye bread
a few dill sprigs

WRAPS

2 large wholemeal tortilla wraps
bunch of watercress
2 cooked beetroots, finely sliced

Break the smoked trout into small pieces, removing any bones, and put them in a bowl. In another bowl, mix the crème fraiche with the horseradish. Add the cucumber and dill to the trout, then fold in the crème fraiche and horseradish mixture. Taste and season with pepper and, if you think it needs it, a squeeze of lemon juice.

If you are having this as a dip, purée or mash until it is quite smooth and serve with sticks of carrot, celery and cucumber.

To make open sandwiches, put a layer of beetroot on slices of bread and top with the trout mixture. Garnish with a few sprigs of dill.

To make wraps, cover each tortilla wrap with sprigs of watercress, then follow with the beetroot. Pile the trout mixture on top. Fold up the bottom of each wrap to stop everything falling out, then roll the whole thing up tightly. Cut the filled wrap in half on the diagonal. If you are not using immediately, wrap it in foil or baking paper for later.

TUNA AND CAPER DIP OR FILLING

A can of tuna is a great thing to have in your store cupboard for a quick, nourishing meal. We love this dip to enjoy as it is or to use as a filling in sandwiches and wraps. (*See photo on colour plate G.*)

61 calories per serving (dip)
118 calories per open sandwich
236 calories per wrap
Makes 4 servings of dip, 4 open sandwiches or 2 wraps

---

1 can of tuna in spring water
juice of 1 lime
2 tbsp light mayonnaise
1 tbsp reduced-fat crème fraiche
a dash of Tabasco
1 tbsp capers, chopped
¼ red pepper, finely chopped
2 spring onions, finely chopped
2 tbsp coriander, finely chopped

OPEN SANDWICHES

¼ **cucumber**

pinch of sugar

1 tsp white wine vinegar

4 slices of wholemeal or rye bread

WRAPS

2 large wholemeal wraps

2 large lettuce leaves, shredded

¼ cucumber, finely sliced lengthways

handful of mint

Drain the tuna and put it in a food processor with the lime juice, mayonnaise and crème fraiche and blitz until smooth. Tip the mixture into a bowl and stir in the rest of the ingredients. Serve as a dip with sticks of carrot and cucumber or pile into lettuce leaves.

To make open sandwiches, slice the cucumber as thinly as you can. Dissolve a pinch of sugar in the vinegar and a tablespoon of water and pour this over the cucumber. Toss lightly, then drain. Put the cucumber on the bread and top with the tuna.

To make wraps, cover each wrap with lettuce, then follow with slices of cucumber. Put the tuna mix on top, then add the mint. Fold up the bottom of each wrap to stop everything falling out, then roll the whole thing up tightly. Cut the wrap in half on the diagonal and serve.

ARTICHOKE AND LEMON DIP

Those roasted artichokes in oil you can buy from the deli counter or in jars are just right for this – better than the ones in brine – but you do have to drain and rinse them thoroughly to keep the cal count down. You still get a nice creamy dip that makes a great snack with some cucumber, celery and other raw veg. This is a lifesaver for those snack-attack moments. (*See photo on colour plate F.*)

50 calories per 50g serving

200g roasted artichokes
grated zest of 1 lemon
juice of ½ lemon
1 garlic clove, crushed
small bunch of basil, leaves only
15g Parmesan cheese, grated
150g reduced-fat crème fraiche
freshly ground black pepper

Drain the roasted artichokes and rinse them thoroughly as the oil will add calories.

Put the artichokes in a food processor with the remaining ingredients and season well with pepper. Blitz until the mixture is fairly smooth – it's good to keep a little texture, but you don't want the dip to be lumpy or fibrous. You may need to push the mixture down with a spatula a couple of times.

Cover and store the dip in the fridge until needed. It will keep well for a couple of days.

LIL'S ROAST
VEGETABLE DIP

Lil, Dave's wife, makes this lush dip, which is called zacusca in Romania and is an Eastern European classic. We've adapted it slightly, reducing the amount of oil to keep the calorie count nice and low, and adding paprika instead of fresh pimentos. We think you're going to love it. Do use fresh tomatoes – they really make a difference here. Serve this dip with raw veg or the socca on page 88. (*See photo on colour plate F.*)

15 calories per 50g serving

---

1 aubergine
1 red pepper, deseeded and halved
1 tbsp olive oil
1 onion, finely chopped
2 garlic cloves, finely grated or crushed
1 tsp sweet smoked paprika
¼ tsp hot smoked paprika
150g ripe tomatoes, peeled and finely chopped
1 bay leaf
1 piece of thinly pared lemon zest (optional)
freshly ground black pepper

Preheat the oven to 220°C/Fan 200°C/Gas 7. Make a few holes in the aubergine and place it on a baking tray with the red pepper. Roast the aubergine and pepper in the preheated oven for 35–40 minutes, turning the aubergine over once or twice, until the skin is blackened. Remove them from the oven. Cut the aubergine in half and leave it to drain for a few minutes. Put the red pepper halves in a bowl and cover, then when they're cool enough to handle, peel off the skin.

Meanwhile, heat the oil in a saucepan. Add the onion with a splash of water, then cover the pan and cook the onion over a low heat for about 10 minutes until soft, stirring regularly.

Add the garlic and paprikas to the onion in the pan and cook for another couple of minutes. Finely chop the aubergine and red pepper and add them to the onions along with the tomatoes. Season with plenty of pepper. Tuck in a bay leaf and lemon zest, if using, then simmer, covered, for half an hour. Uncover and continue to cook, stirring regularly, until thick.

If you want a smoother dip, purée it in a blender or food processor – take out the bay leaf and lemon zest first. Leave the dip to cool down and serve at room temperature.

BIKER TIP

To peel fresh tomatoes, score a cross in the base of each one. Put them in a bowl, pour over freshly boiled water and count to 10, then drain. The skin will peel off very easily.

SOCCA AND SALSA

Sounds like a new dance! These chickpea flour flatbreads, known as socca, are addictive. Enjoy with the salsa or one of the dips in this chapter. (*See photo on colour plate G.*)

262 calories per serving
Serves 4

---

2 tbsp olive oil
2 red onions, thinly sliced into wedges
150g chickpea (gram) flour
low-cal olive oil spray
1 tsp finely chopped rosemary
freshly ground black pepper

SALSA
4 tomatoes, cored and diced
½ small red onion, finely chopped
1 small red chilli, finely chopped
zest of ½ lemon
1 tsp red wine vinegar
1 tsp olive oil
small bunch of basil, finely chopped

UNDER 220 CALORIES

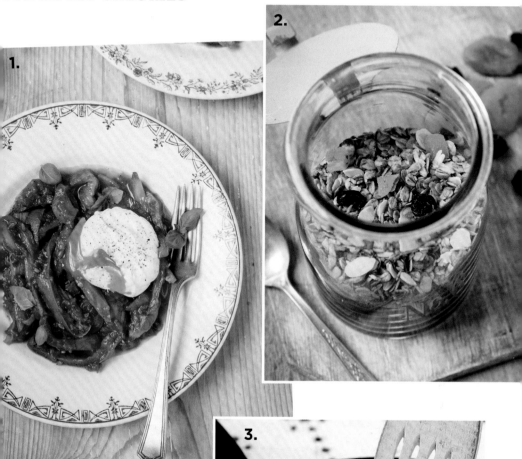

1. Mediterranean Biker brunch
   (153 cals, p.28)

2. Stove-top granola
   (213 cals, p.16)

3. Buckwheat pancakes with
   eggs and mushrooms
   (193 cals, p.32)

BREAKFAST AND BRUNCH

UNDER 300 CALORIES

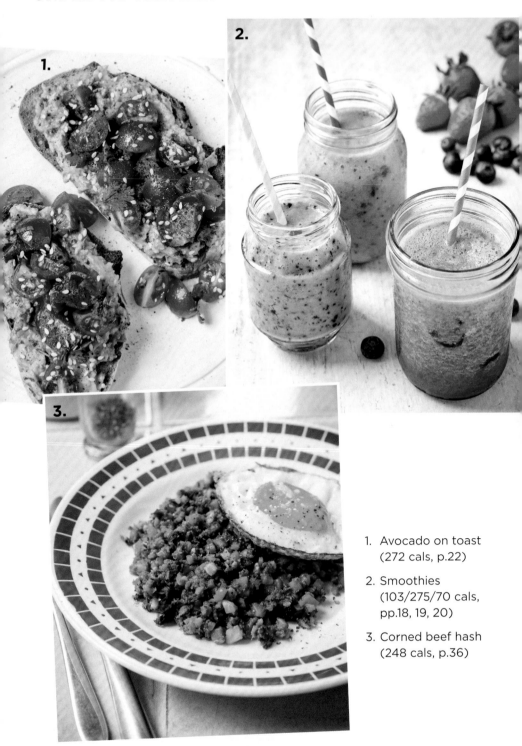

1. Avocado on toast
   (272 cals, p.22)

2. Smoothies
   (103/275/70 cals,
   pp.18, 19, 20)

3. Corned beef hash
   (248 cals, p.36)

UNDER 200 CALORIES

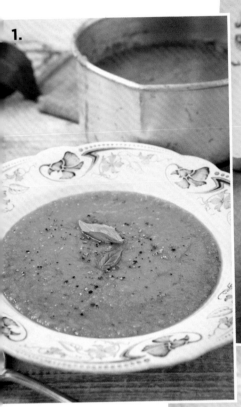

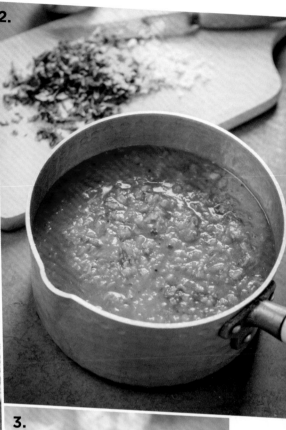

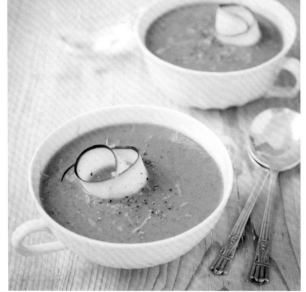

1. Tomato soup
   (171 cals, p.42)

2. Red lentil and harissa
   soup (166 cals, p.48)

3. Courgette, mint and
   lemon soup
   (105 cals, p.46)

SOUPS

UNDER 300 CALORIES

1. Bean and vegetable soup
   (290 cals, p.50)

2. Pea, lettuce and asparagus
   soup (220 cals, p.44)

3. Scotch broth
   (240 cals, p.56)

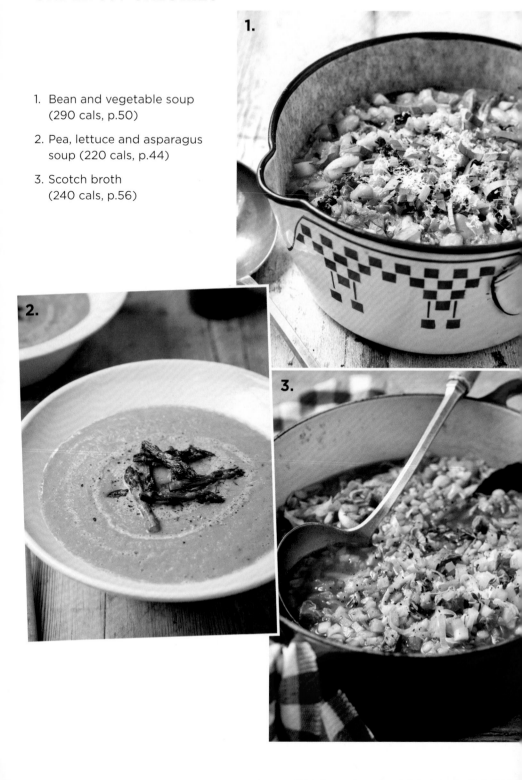

SALADS

UNDER 200 CALORIES

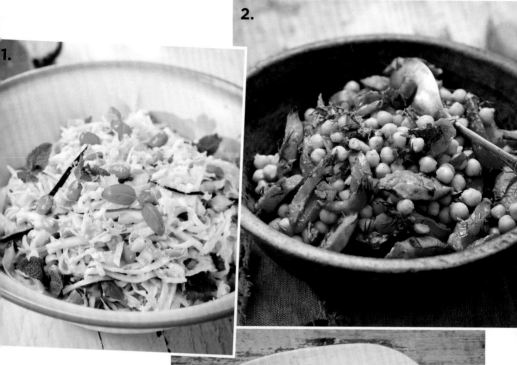

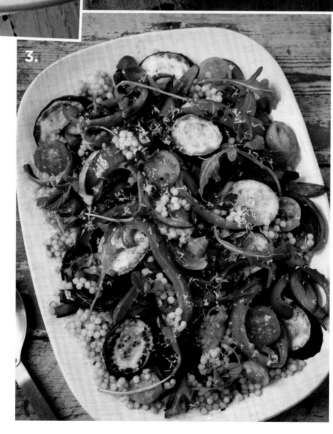

1. Summery green
coleslaw
(130 cals, p.60)

2. Roasted carrot, pepper
and chickpea salad
(136 cals, p.58)

3. Harissa vegetables and
jumbo couscous
(197 cals, p.64)

SNACKS AND DIPS

UNDER 60 CALORIES

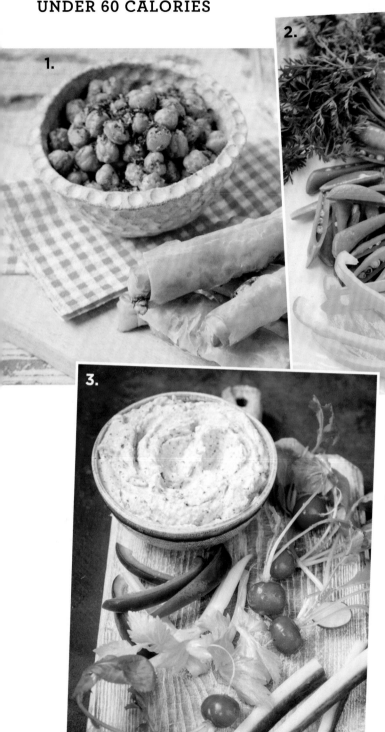

1 Roast chickpeas
   (40 cals, p.90)

2. Lil's roast vegetable
   dip (15 cals, p.86)

3. Artichoke and lemon
   dip (50 cals, p.84)

UNDER 250 CALORIES

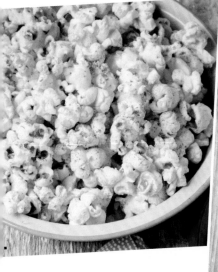

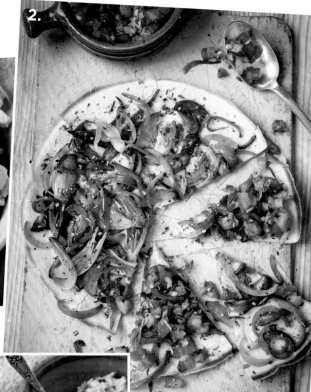

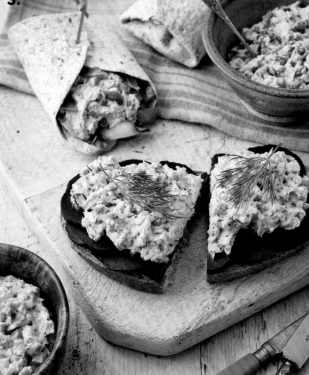

1 Spiced popcorn
   (81 cals, p.92)

2. Socca and salsa
   (262 cals, p.88)

3. Smoked trout dip
   or filling (58/146/
   157 cals, p.80), and
   Tuna and caper dip
   or filling (61/118/
   236 cals, p.82)

VEGGIE TREATS

UNDER 200 CALORIES

1. Bubble and squeak
   (107/195 cals, p.130)

2. Thai vegetable curry
   (170 cals, p.102)

3. Vegetable curry
   (91 cals, p.114)

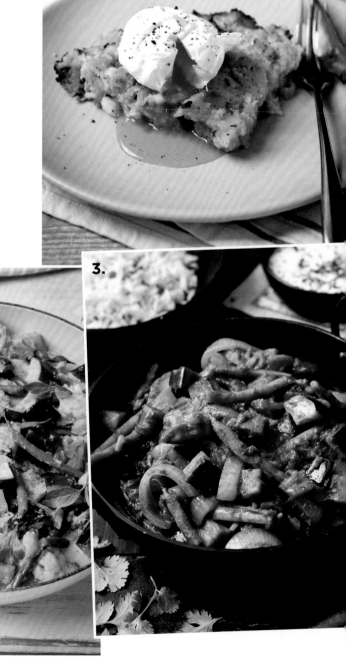

Heat a tablespoon of the oil in a frying pan and add the red onions. Fry them over a medium heat for at least 10 minutes until they have softened and started to caramelise. Set aside.

Put the chickpea flour in a bowl and whisk to remove any lumps. Gradually pour in 250ml of water and continue to whisk until you have a smooth batter with the consistency of thick double cream. Stir in the remaining olive oil and whisk to emulsify. Set the batter aside.

To make the salsa, mix all the ingredients together in a bowl and season well with pepper.

You can make 2 large socca in a 25cm non-stick pan, or 4 in a smaller pan. If making 2 large socca, heat the pan and spritz with oil. Pour half the batter into the pan and swirl to cover the base. Sprinkle over half the onions and half the rosemary, then cook over a medium heat for a few minutes until browned and crisping round the edges. Flip the socca over to cook the other side or put the pan under a medium grill to finish the cooking. Transfer it to a board or a large plate and repeat.

If you are cooking 4 socca, split the batter into 4 and proceed as above, using a quarter of the onions and rosemary each time. Cut the socca into wedges or serve whole with the salsa.

ROAST CHICKPEAS

These make a cracking good snack without too many calories, as long as you keep to a sensible portion of course! Sumac is a lovely lemony spice, but you can use some chilli or paprika instead if you prefer or you don't have sumac. (*See photo on colour plate F.*)

40 calories per 25g serving

400g can of chickpeas, drained and rinsed
1 tbsp olive oil
zest of 1 lemon
½ tsp rosemary
1 tsp sumac
freshly ground black pepper

Preheat the oven to 200°C/Fan 180°C/Gas 6. First dry the chickpeas by wrapping them in a tea towel, or by gently blotting them with kitchen paper, then put them in a bowl. Drizzle over the olive oil, then add the lemon zest and a generous amount of black pepper.

Spread the chickpeas over a baking tray and roast them in the oven for 25–30 minutes. Check them regularly and give the tray a shake so the chickpeas roast evenly. The chickpeas are done when they are nicely browned and crisp on the outside, but still soft on the inside.

Transfer the chickpeas to a bowl, then add the rosemary and sumac and stir. Great hot or cold.

SPICED POPCORN

Like everyone, we love popcorn, and if you make your own at home you can be sure it's not packed with sugar and salt. This is a good low-cal snack that's both satisfying and healthy. (*See photo on colour plate G.*)

81 calories per serving

Serves 4

---

1 tsp vegetable oil

75g popping corn

1 tsp mild chilli powder

zest of 1 lime

1 tsp salt (optional)

1 tbsp lime juice

Heat the oil in a large lidded saucepan. Add the popping corn and put the lid on the pan. Cook over a medium heat for about 4-5 minutes, shaking regularly when the corn starts popping while holding down the lid.

When the popping has stopped completely (when you go for about 15 seconds without hearing any sound), it will be safe to remove the lid. Tip the popcorn into a bowl, discarding any kernels that haven't popped.

Mix the chilli powder, lime zest and salt, if using, together. Shake this mixture over the popcorn, making sure it is all well dusted, then sprinkle over the lime juice.

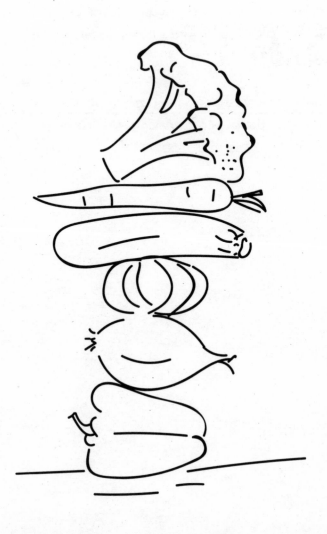

VEGGIE
TREATS

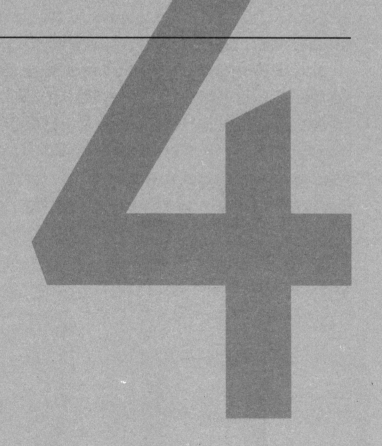

Whether or not you want to go totally vegetarian, it's a good idea to cut down on your meat intake. Aim to have several meat-free days every week and make your meals from delicious vegetables, pulses and wholegrains. If you do have diabetes, it's important to be a healthy weight or you can be at greater risk of heart disease. Research shows that people who have a mainly or totally vegetarian diet are less likely to be overweight or to suffer from heart disease or high blood pressure, so getting your five a day is helpful all round. If you're worried about getting enough protein without meat, don't be. There's plenty of protein in lovely plant-based foods, such as nuts, seeds, beans and lentils.

Baked potatoes with broccoli and cheese 98

Barley risotto with greens 100

Thai vegetable curry 102

Aubergine bake 106

Roast vegetable lasagne 110

Vegetable curry 114

Black-eyed beans and greens 116

Vegetarian pasta 118

Green pasta 120

Latin American shepherd's pie 122

Cauliflower and broccoli cheese 126

Pesto-stuffed mushrooms 128

Bubble and squeak 130

Grilled aubergines with chickpea
and spinach salad 134

BAKED POTATOES WITH BROCCOLI AND CHEESE

Baked potatoes have long been – and always will be – a go-to supper for us. And this simple but delicious filling makes the humble spud into a guilt-free meal to be proud of. (*See photo on colour plate J.*)

274 calories per serving (white potatoes)
289 calories per serving (sweet potatoes)
Serves 4

---

4 baking potatoes or sweet potatoes, well scrubbed and
   patted dry
low-cal olive oil spray

FILLING
350g broccoli, cut into very small florets and thicker stems
   sliced
75g reduced-fat vegetarian cheese, grated
25g quark
1 tsp wholegrain mustard
freshly ground black pepper

For baking potatoes, preheat the oven to 200°C/Fan 180°C/ Gas 6. Cut a deep cross in each potato and pierce it all over with a fork. Spritz with oil, then bake for 60–75 minutes until cooked through. Squeeze each potato from the bottom so that the cut cross opens out. Top with the filling.

For sweet potatoes, preheat the oven to 180°C/Fan 160°C/ Gas 4. Pierce each potato all over with a fork, then place the potatoes on a baking tray. Spritz with olive oil then roast for 50–60 minutes until cooked. Split and top with the filling.

To make the filling, bring a large pan of water to the boil. Boil the broccoli for 3–4 minutes or until just tender, then drain. Put the cheese in a small pan with the quark and mustard. Stir over a low heat until the cheese has melted into a sauce. Fold in the broccoli and season with pepper.

BARLEY RISOTTO WITH GREENS

Barley makes a great risotto and is a nice change from rice. It's packed full of minerals and vitamins too, so let's eat more of it. You can also make this tasty dish with spelt if you fancy. (*See photo on colour plate J.*)

322 calories per serving (without cheese)
348 calories per serving (with cheese)
Serves 4

---

1 tsp olive oil

10g butter

1 onion, finely chopped

2 garlic cloves, finely chopped

1 tsp fresh thyme leaves

zest of 1 lemon

200g pearl barley, rinsed

100ml white wine

1 litre vegetable stock

400g tenderstem or sprouting broccoli

100g runner beans, shredded, or broad beans

100g peas

freshly ground black pepper

To finish

25g vegetarian Parmesan-style hard cheese, grated (optional)
handful of basil leaves, torn

Heat the olive oil and butter in a saucepan, then add the onion and cook it over a gentle heat for a few minutes until it's starting to soften. Add the garlic and cook for another minute, then add the thyme, lemon zest and barley. Stir until the grains look glossy, then pour over the wine. Bring it to the boil and let most of the wine boil off, then pour in the stock. Season with black pepper.

Bring the stock to the boil, then turn the heat down and simmer gently, stirring regularly to make sure the barley doesn't catch on the bottom of the pan.

Meanwhile, bring a large saucepan of water to the boil. Trim the broccoli and cut it into chunks, then add it to the pan with beans and simmer for 2 minutes. Add the peas and cook for another minute, then drain everything into a colander.

When most of the liquid has been absorbed by the barley, check the texture – if the grains aren't quite done, add a little more liquid if necessary. When you are happy the barley is cooked, beat in the cheese, if using, then fold in all the greens. Garnish with basil leaves and serve.

THAI VEGETABLE CURRY

Obviously you can use shop-bought curry paste if you prefer but our home-made version is quick to make and tastes fantastic. We've included Thai basil, which you see in lots of supermarkets now, but don't worry too much if you don't have any. Just use a mix of ordinary basil and coriander instead. (*See photo on colour plate H.*)

170 calories per serving
Serves 4

---

1 tsp vegetable oil
2 shallots, thinly sliced
400ml reduced-fat coconut milk
200ml hot vegetable stock
2 Kaffir lime leaves, shredded
1 medium aubergine
200g butternut squash
200g green beans
1 large courgette
½ small cauliflower (about 200g)
juice of 1 lime
small bunch of coriander leaves, to serve
small bunch of Thai basil (optional), to serve
freshly ground black pepper

CURRY PASTE

1 red chilli

1 tbsp coriander stems

2 shallots

4 garlic cloves

10g chunk of fresh root ginger

2 lemongrass stalks or 1 tbsp lemongrass paste

1 tbsp galangal paste (optional)

1 tbsp soy sauce or tamari

½ tsp turmeric

First prepare the ingredients for the curry paste. Deseed the chilli if you want to decrease the heat. Roughly chop the chilli, coriander stems, shallots and garlic. Peel and chop the ginger. Remove the outer layers of the lemongrass stalks, if using, then roughly chop the soft white centres.

Put all the paste ingredients into a food processor with some pepper. Add a splash of water and blitz until fairly smooth.

Put the oil in a large pan. Add the shallots and cook them for a couple of minutes, then add the paste. Stir the paste for 2–3 minutes until it smells very aromatic, then pour in the coconut milk and vegetable stock. Add the lime leaves, season with pepper and leave to simmer gently while you prepare the rest of the ingredients.

CONTINUED ON NEXT PAGE

Cut the aubergine and butternut squash into fairly large chunks of about 3cm. Add them to the pan, cover the pan with a lid and simmer for 5 minutes. Meanwhile, trim the green beans, cut the courgette into chunks and separate the cauliflower into florets, cutting them in half if very large. Add these to the pan, then cover again and simmer for a further 5 minutes.

When all the vegetables are tender, add the lime juice. Taste the curry for seasoning and add more soy sauce or tamari if you think it needs it. Serve sprinkled with coriander leaves and Thai basil leaves, if using.

Vegetables and fruit are your best friends if you have type 2 diabetes. Try to make sure you always have your five portions a day – we do!

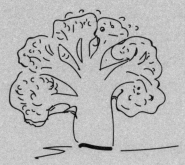

AUBERGINE BAKE

Our low-cal version of an Italian classic – melanzane parmigiana – makes a comforting and delicious supper dish. There's lots of oil in the traditional version, but we've cut back on that to keep the calories down, while making sure there's still plenty of tasty sauce. Use one or two balls of mozzarella as you like, but remember that more mozz means more calories. Check that your mozzarella is suitable for vegetarians.

205 calories per serving
(with one ball of mozzarella)
269 calories per serving
(with two balls of mozzarella)
Serves 4

---

4 large aubergines, sliced into 1cm rounds
low-cal olive oil spray
handful of basil leaves, torn
1 or 2 balls of half-fat mozzarella

TOMATO SAUCE
1 tbsp olive oil
1 onion, finely chopped
2 garlic cloves, finely chopped

1 tsp oregano

small pinch of cinnamon

small pinch of sugar

200ml red wine

2 x 400g cans of chopped tomatoes

freshly ground black pepper

Preheat the oven to 200°C/Fan 180°C/Gas 6. You may need to cook the aubergines in a couple of batches. Line 2 large baking trays with non-stick baking paper. Arrange the slices of aubergine on the trays, then mist them very lightly with oil – you will probably need about 3 sprays per tray.

Put the baking trays in the oven and roast the aubergine slices until they are soft and the flesh is golden brown in patches. This will take about 40–45 minutes. Remove the aubergines from the oven and set them aside to cool while you cook the rest of the slices in the same way.

Meanwhile, make the tomato sauce. Heat the olive oil in a large saucepan. Add the onion and fry over a low heat until soft and translucent. Add the garlic and cook for another 2 minutes. Sprinkle over the oregano, cinnamon and sugar and give everything a quick stir.

Pour in the red wine and turn up the heat, then simmer quite briskly until the liquid has reduced by about half. Add the

CONTINUED ON NEXT PAGE

tomatoes and season with pepper, then simmer for at least 20 minutes, until the sauce has reduced and thickened.

Take a large ovenproof baking dish and spread a little of the tomato sauce on the bottom. Cover with a layer of aubergines and some roughly torn basil, then continue adding layers of sauce and aubergines until you have used everything up – you should have at least 3 layers of aubergines. Finish with a thin layer of tomato sauce.

Slice the mozzarella as thinly as you can and arrange it over the aubergines and sauce. It doesn't matter if there are gaps, it will spread a little during cooking. Put the dish in the oven and bake for 30 minutes until the aubergines are very tender and the mozzarella has melted and browned a little. Serve with a green salad.

Aubergines have a chunky, meaty feel but they're reassuringly low in calories, so good for filling you up without bulking you up.

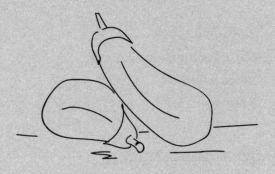

ROAST VEGETABLE LASAGNE

Make this the regular way or replace the sheets of pasta with leek leaves. Either way it tastes fantastic and is a real treat for the family. Even the pasta version isn't too high in calories for such a satisfying dish.

241 calories per serving (with leeks)
343 calories per serving (with dried lasagne)
Serves 6

---

1 aubergine, halved lengthways and cut into crescents
200g piece of pumpkin or squash, sliced into thin wedges
1 large red onion, cut into thin wedges
2 red peppers and 1 green pepper, deseeded and halved
1 garlic bulb, cloves separated but unpeeled
1 tsp dried oregano
low-cal olive oil spray
freshly ground black pepper

Béchamel sauce
600ml semi-skimmed milk
1 slice of onion
2 cloves

1 bay leaf
20g cornflour
white pepper

To assemble
2 large leeks, trimmed or 150g dried wholewheat lasagne
1 quantity of tomato sauce (see page 208)
50g reduced-fat vegetarian Cheddar cheese, grated
25g vegetarian Parmesan-style hard cheese, grated

Preheat the oven to 200°C/Fan 180°C/Gas 6. Arrange the aubergine, pumpkin or squash, onion, peppers and garlic over 2 roasting tins or trays. Sprinkle with the oregano and spritz with oil. Roast the vegetables for 25–30 minutes until they are charred in places and just cooked through, then remove them from the oven.

Squeeze the flesh from the garlic cloves and chop it roughly. Put the peppers in a bowl and cover. When they are cool enough to handle, skin them and cut the flesh into strips.

If using pasta, cook it according to the packet instructions. If using leeks, trim them to the same width as your lasagne dish. Cut them through the middle, then take the larger leaves from the outside of the leeks. Bring a large pot of water to the boil, add the leek leaves and simmer them for 5 minutes or until

CONTINUED ON NEXT PAGE

very tender. Drain the leaves and cool them under cold running water, then lay them out on kitchen paper or a clean tea towel to absorb any excess liquid.

To make the béchamel sauce, put the milk in a pan with the slice of onion, cloves and bay leaf. Heat until the milk is just coming up to the boil, then remove the pan from the heat and leave the milk to infuse until it's almost cold.

Strain the milk into a jug, rinse out the pan, then pour the milk back into it. Mix the cornflour with a little cold water to make a smooth, thin paste. Reheat the milk and pour in the paste. Gradually bring the sauce to the boil, stirring constantly. When the sauce is the consistency of double cream, season it with white pepper and set aside.

To assemble the lasagne, spoon half the tomato sauce over your lasagne dish and top with half the roasted vegetables. Spoon over a little of the béchamel sauce and top with leek leaves or pasta sheets, making sure everything is covered. Repeat this until you have used up all the tomato sauce, vegetables and leek or pasta sheets.

Cover with the remaining béchamel, then sprinkle with the grated cheese. Bake in the oven for 40–45 minutes until the cheese is a rich golden brown and the lasagne is piping hot.

It's worth making a big batch of tomato sauce and stashing some in the freezer. It's great for quick pasta suppers and makes coming up with a delicious lasagne a lot quicker and easier.

VEGETABLE CURRY

There's more fibre in this veggie treat than in a brillo pad and it's much tastier of course! Vegetable curries, especially those with aubergine, often contain lots of oil. We've kept the amount of oil down by cooking the aubergine on a fairly high heat so it seals quickly and doesn't soak up too much. Serve with rice or flatbread if you like. (*See photo on colour plate H.*)

91 calories per serving
Serves 4

---

1 tbsp vegetable oil

1 tsp cumin seeds

1 onion, thickly sliced

1 aubergine, diced

200g mushrooms, wiped and halved

1 courgette, diced

2 garlic cloves, finely chopped

10g chunk of fresh root ginger, peeled and grated

1 tbsp medium curry powder

100g green beans, halved

400g can of tomatoes

large handful of fresh coriander leaves

freshly ground black pepper

To serve

4 tbsp fat-free natural yoghurt

1 tsp dried mint (optional)

Heat the oil in a large frying pan and add the cumin seeds, onion, aubergine, mushrooms and courgette. Cook the vegetables over a medium heat, stirring regularly, until they have started to soften around the edges and have taken on a bit of colour.

Add the garlic and ginger, then sprinkle over the curry powder and season with pepper. Add the green beans and pour in 200ml of water. Simmer for 2 minutes, then add the tomatoes. Simmer for about 20 minutes, until the vegetables are tender and the curry has thickened.

Just before serving, stir in a handful of fresh coriander. Serve with yoghurt and stir in some dried mint into it if you like.

BLACK-EYED BEANS AND GREENS

We love the food of the southern US and this is our version of a Cajun favourite – black-eyed peas and greens. We call 'em black-eyed beans over here but they're the same thing.

207 calories per serving
Serves 4

---

1 tbsp vegetable oil

1 white onion, diced

2 celery sticks, diced

1 green pepper, deseeded and diced

2 tsp garlic powder

1 tsp onion powder (optional)

1 tsp sweet smoked paprika

1 tsp ground cumin

½ tsp cayenne pepper

1 tsp dried oregano or mixed herbs

2 bay leaves

2 x 400g cans of black-eyed beans, drained and rinsed

500ml hot vegetable stock

200g spring greens

freshly ground black pepper

Heat the oil in a large pan over a medium heat. Add the onion, celery and green pepper to the pan, turn the heat up to high and stir for 5 minutes – the vegetables should be browning nicely by this point.

Sprinkle over the garlic powder and onion powder, if using, and the spices and herbs. Stir for a minute, and then add the beans. Pour over the vegetable stock and season with pepper.

Bring to the boil, cover the pan, then turn down the heat and cook for 5 minutes. During this time, wash and shred the spring greens. Pile these on top of the beans, but do not stir at this stage.

Turn the heat up again and cover the pan. After 5 minutes the spring greens will have wilted down a little. Stir to combine with the rest of the ingredients and leave to simmer for a further 5 minutes before serving.

VEGETARIAN PASTA

This pasta dish freezes and reheats well so it's worth making a big batch and storing some in the freezer for another day. You can double up the quantities if you like. It's perfect for the unexpected guest – they'll be well impressed. (*See photo on colour plate J.*)

290 calories per serving
Serves 4

---

2 tsp olive oil

1 onion, finely chopped

1 celery stick, finely chopped

2 garlic cloves, finely chopped

1 large courgette, diced

1 tsp dried rosemary, or a sprig of fresh, finely chopped

zest of ½ lemon

200g cavolo nero, shredded

150g broad beans (frozen are fine)

250ml vegetable stock

2 medium tomatoes, peeled and finely chopped

200g short wholewheat pasta, such as farfalle

20g vegetarian Parmesan-style cheese, grated, to serve

freshly ground black pepper

Heat the oil in a pan, add the onion and celery, then sauté them over a medium heat until they're nicely soft and translucent. Add the garlic and courgette and cook for another couple of minutes.

Sprinkle over the rosemary and lemon zest, then add the cavolo nero and broad beans. Pour over the stock, add the tomatoes, then simmer, uncovered, until the liquid has reduced by two-thirds and the vegetables are tender. Season with black pepper.

Meanwhile, bring a large pan of water to the boil, add the pasta and cook until just al dente – cooked but with a little bite to it. Drain the pasta and toss it with the sauce to combine. Serve with a little grated cheese.

BIKER TIP

If you freeze this dish, let it defrost naturally, then put it in a saucepan with a splash of water. Cover the pan and warm the pasta through over a low heat.

GREEN PASTA

Pasta and pesto is one of our favourite suppers, but the regular version contains lots of oil, cheese and nuts so is quite rich. Try our healthier, lighter recipe, which cuts down the calories, but not the flavour, and uses a little of the pasta cooking water to thicken the sauce – a classic Italian tip. This is super-quick to make and great warm, or cool as a salad. Makes a great lunch-box treat too. (*See photo on colour plate l.*)

239 calories per serving

Serves 4

200g short wholewheat pasta
1 large courgette, grated
large bunch of basil
1 garlic clove, finely chopped
1 tbsp olive oil
grated zest of 1 lemon
25g vegetarian Parmesan-style cheese, grated
freshly ground black pepper

Bring a large pan of water to the boil, add the pasta and cook for 10–12 minutes, or until cooked through but still with a bit of bite to it. Add the grated courgette at the last minute.

Put the basil, garlic, oil and lemon zest in a food processor with a small ladleful of the cooking liquor – do this towards the end of the cooking time so the water will have more starch in it. Season with pepper, then blitz the sauce until it's fairly smooth but still flecked with green from the basil.

Drain the pasta and courgette, toss it with the sauce and serve with grated cheese.

LATIN AMERICAN SHEPHERD'S PIE

This is a winner. Everyone's favourite, a good old shepherd's pie but with a tasty chilli twist and a sweetcorn topping instead of mashed potatoes. Make this and it won't just be the pie that's full of beans. The filling is a delight of spicy loveliness, but there isn't a lot of topping – we're keeping the calories down – so use a fairly deep dish so you don't have to spread the topping too thinly.

400 calories per serving (4)
266 calories per serving (6)
Serves 4-6

---

1 large red onion
2 celery sticks
1 large carrot
1 red pepper and 1 green pepper, deseeded
1 tsp vegetable oil
2 garlic cloves, chopped
1 tbsp ground cumin
1 tsp ground coriander
½ tsp cinnamon
½ tsp smoked chilli powder (chipotle)

2 tbsp finely chopped coriander stems

400g can of kidney beans

400g can of butter beans

400g can of tomatoes

300ml vegetable stock

freshly ground black pepper

TOPPING

500g sweetcorn kernels

3 tbsp fine cornmeal (polenta) or plain flour

1 tsp baking powder

15g butter

50g reduced-fat vegetarian Cheddar, grated

Finely chop the onion and celery sticks and dice the carrot and peppers.

Heat the oil in a large pan and add all the vegetables, along with a splash of water. Cover the pan and leave the vegetables to cook gently until soft – this should take about 15 minutes. Add the garlic, spices and chopped coriander stems and then stir to combine.

Add all the beans, then pour over the tomatoes and the stock. Season with pepper, then bring everything to the boil. Reduce the heat and leave to simmer until the sauce is well reduced,

CONTINUED ON NEXT PAGE

then tip everything into a deep oven dish. Preheat the oven to 190°C/Fan 170°C/Gas 5.

To make the topping, put half the sweetcorn kernels in a food processor with the cornmeal or flour, baking powder and butter, then blitz until smooth. Season with plenty of pepper, then add the remaining sweetcorn and blitz again to make a mixture with a rough, dropping consistency.

Spread the topping evenly over the filling and sprinkle with the grated cheese. Bake the pie in the oven for 30–40 minutes until the topping is a deep golden-brown and the filling is piping hot.

You need to cut down on salt if you have type 2 diabetes, so use lots of lovely herbs in your cooking and you will have great flavour without the risk factors.

CAULIFLOWER AND BROCCOLI CHEESE

Cauli cheese is a big warm cuddle of a dish. We've adapted this favourite by adding extra flavours to the sauce and reducing the amount of cheese to make it less calorific. And the mix of broccoli and cauliflower makes the dish look really special. Some roasted tomatoes go well with this. *(See photo on colour plate I.)*

261 calories per serving
Serves 4

600ml semi-skimmed milk

1 slice of onion

2 cloves

1 bay leaf

1 cauliflower (500–600g, trimmed weight), broken into florets

1 head of broccoli (about 300g), broken into florets

20g cornflour

1 heaped tsp wholegrain mustard

50g reduced-fat vegetarian Cheddar, grated

2 tbsp finely chopped parsley

freshly ground black pepper

TOPPING

25g reduced-fat vegetarian Cheddar, finely grated
1 tbsp fine wholemeal breadcrumbs

Pour the milk in a pan and add the onion, cloves and bay leaf. Heat until the milk is just coming up to the boil, then remove the pan from the heat and leave the milk to infuse while you cook the vegetables.

Bring a large pan of water to the boil. Add the cauliflower and cook for 3 minutes, then add the broccoli to the pan and cook for another 2 minutes. Check for doneness. The cauliflower and broccoli should be tender but still have a little bite to them – al dente, as they say. Drain the vegetables thoroughly and put them in a large ovenproof dish. Preheat the oven to 200°C/Fan 180°C/Gas 6.

Strain the milk into a jug, then rinse out the saucepan and pour the milk back in. Mix the cornflour with a little cold water in a bowl and stir until you have a smooth, thin paste. Put the pan of milk back over the heat and pour in the cornflour mixture. Gradually bring the sauce to the boil, stirring constantly until it has thickened. Add the mustard, cheese and parsley to the sauce, season with pepper and stir until the cheese has melted. Pour the sauce over the cauliflower and broccoli.

Mix the cheese and breadcrumbs together to make the topping and sprinkle it over the sauce. Bake in the oven for 20–25 minutes until well browned and bubbling. Fantastic!

PESTO-STUFFED MUSHROOMS

Someone used to say that life is too short to stuff a mushroom, but we disagree when it comes to these little beauties! These don't take too long to put to together and make a really satisfying dish with the butter beans and spinach. (*See photo on colour plate I.*)

209 calories per serving
Serves 4

---

4 large field or Portobello mushrooms, wiped clean

25g panko breadcrumbs

1 large courgette, diagonally sliced

low-cal olive oil spray

1 tbsp tomato purée

1 tsp dried oregano

400g can of butter beans, drained

100g spinach, washed

PESTO

50g fresh basil, leaves only

30g vegetarian Parmesan-style cheese, grated

25g pine nuts

zest and juice of 1 lemon
1 tbsp olive oil
freshly ground black pepper

Preheat the oven to 200°C/Fan 180°C/Gas 6.

To make the pesto, put all the ingredients in a small food processor and season with pepper. Blitz to make a coarse paste, stopping to push down the ingredients in the bowl and adding a little water if necessary.

Place the mushrooms in a roasting tin, undersides facing up. Spread a tablespoon of pesto over each mushroom and top with some breadcrumbs. Add the courgette slices in between the mushrooms and spritz them with oil. Put the tin in the oven and roast the mushrooms for 10 minutes.

Mix the tomato purée and oregano with 100ml of water in a bowl and stir in the butter beans. Take the tin out of the oven and add the butter bean mixture around the mushrooms. Take care that the liquid doesn't go over the mushrooms – it's fine for it to cover the courgettes. Cook for a further 20 minutes.

Remove the tin from the oven. Arrange the spinach over 4 plates and top with the stuffed mushrooms, courgettes and butter beans.

BUBBLE AND SQUEAK

There's nothing like a good bubble – it's a great favourite of ours. In this recipe we've upped the carrot and swede and cut down on the potato so it's a bit lighter than usual but still tastes mega. Swede can go a bit mushy when boiled, so we like to steam the veg, but if you don't have a steamer, just be sure to drain it all well. You could dry-fry the eggs instead of poaching them, if you prefer. (*See photo on colour plate H.*)

107 calories per serving
195 calories per serving (with poached egg)
Serves 4

200g swede, peeled and diced
200g carrots, peeled and diced
200g potatoes, peeled and diced
200g cabbage, shredded
1 tsp olive oil
½ onion, finely chopped
4 eggs (optional)
1 tsp white wine vinegar (optional)
freshly ground black pepper

Layer the root vegetables in a steamer – swede on the bottom, carrots next, potatoes on top. Steam them over boiling water for 10 minutes or until all the vegetables are tender. If you don't have a steamer, boil the vegetables until tender, then drain them really well.

Season the veg with pepper and then mash. You don't want the mixture to be too smooth, so don't be too vigorous.

Put the cabbage in a saucepan with a couple of centimetres of just-boiled water and simmer it for a few minutes until tender. Drain thoroughly. Add the olive oil to a large non-stick frying pan and fry the onion until it is translucent and taking on a little colour. Tip the onion into the mash, along with the cabbage, and stir.

Heat the grill to its highest setting. Pile all the mixture into the frying pan and cook over a medium heat for several minutes until you see that it is browning around the edges. Put the pan under the grill until the top has crisped up a bit and is a good deep brown.

If you want to top the mixture with eggs, try our great tip for successful poaching. Half fill a medium non-stick saucepan

CONTINUED ON NEXT PAGE

with water, add a teaspoon of vinegar and bring it to the boil. Place the eggs, still in their shells, into the boiling water for exactly 20 seconds – this helps the whites stay together. Remove them with a slotted spoon and turn the heat down so the water is simmering gently.

Crack the eggs into the water and cook for 3 minutes. The water should be gently bubbling and the eggs will rise to the surface when they are nearly ready. Remove them with a slotted spoon, drain briefly and place an egg on top of each helping of bubble and squeak.

An egg is only between 55 and 80 calories depending on size, and so makes a great protein addition to a veggie meal.

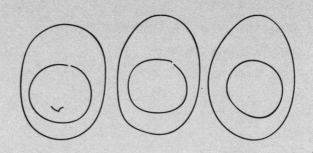

GRILLED AUBERGINES WITH CHICKPEA AND SPINACH SALAD

The aubergines make a great starter just with the yoghurt sauce but they're even better with the chickpea salad too. This is a good vegetarian dish, but check the feta you're using is suitable and not made with animal rennet.

205 calories per serving
Serves 4

---

3 medium aubergines
low-cal olive oil spray
50g vegetarian feta cheese (optional)
freshly ground black pepper

YOGHURT DRESSING
large pinch of saffron
30ml hot water
200g low-fat or 0%-fat Greek yoghurt
1 garlic clove, crushed
1 tsp dried mint

CHICKPEA AND SPINACH SALAD

1 tsp olive oil

1 garlic clove, finely chopped

400g can of chickpeas, drained and rinsed

1 tsp ground cumin

grated zest of 1 lemon

200g fresh baby leaf spinach

Heat the grill to its highest setting. Top and tail the aubergines, making sure you cut at least 1cm away from the top, as this can be a bit tough. Cut the aubergines into ½cm slices. You should get at least 12 good-sized slices from each aubergine, as well as the smaller end bits.

Spritz 2 non-stick baking trays with low-cal oil spray and arrange the aubergine slices on the trays. Spray the aubergines with oil and season them with pepper. Place one of the trays under the grill, preferably on the second shelf down (they will burn if right at the top), then grill the slices for 5 minutes. Turn them over and grill for another 5 minutes or 3 minutes if adding feta.

If using feta, crumble half of it over the grilled aubergine slices, then grill for a further 2 minutes. Remove the tray from the grill, then cook the second batch in the same way.

CONTINUED ON NEXT PAGE

For the salad, heat the oil in a large saucepan and add the garlic. Cook it for a minute, then add the chickpeas, cumin, lemon zest and 50ml of water. Season with pepper and leave to simmer over a low heat until warmed through. Thoroughly wash the spinach and shake it briefly to get rid of any excess water. Add the spinach to the pan, pushing it down as it wilts. Leave it for a couple of minutes to combine with the chickpeas, then stir.

To make the yoghurt dressing, soak the saffron in the hot water for 5 minutes. Whisk the saffron and its soaking liquor into the yoghurt with the garlic and dried mint. Season with pepper and serve with the aubergine slices and the chickpea and spinach salad.

Reducing the amount of fat you eat helps cut calories. Low-fat products are great, but check the ingredients carefully as some are high in sugar.

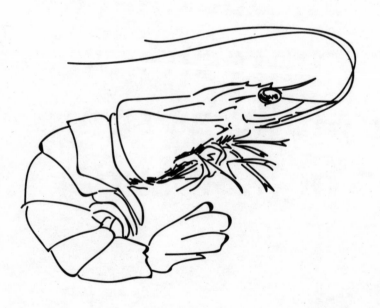

HEARTY
SUPPERS

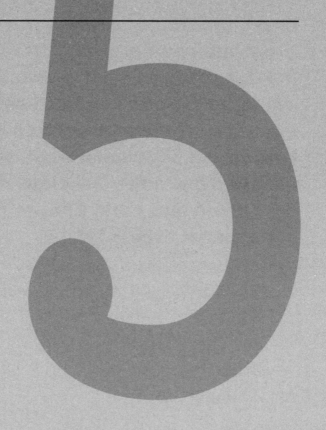

In this chapter we've included plenty of our favourite fish recipes, as fish is a great source of protein and is good for your heart health – important if you're suffering from diabetes. Oily fish, such as salmon, is particularly beneficial because although it is relatively high in calories, it contains a good supply of omega-3 oil, which is beneficial for your heart. Chicken and turkey are another great source of protein and they're low in fat, as long as you remove the skin. We certainly don't need to eat meat every day and we think red meat is best kept for an occasional treat, so we've included just a few delicious recipes for beef, lamb and pork. Choose lean cuts and remove excess fat.

Baked fish with red peppers and tomatoes 142

White bean and tuna fishcakes 144

Mediterranean fish casserole 148

Fish curry 150

Salmon and broccoli tray bake 152

Mackerel fillets with gremolata 154

Fish crumble 158

Chilli prawn pasta 162

Turkey chilli with cauliflower 'rice' 164

Garlic chicken with beans, kale
and cherry tomatoes 168

Fusion tandoori chicken 170

Chicken tray bake with fennel, peas
and new potatoes 172

Caribbean chicken curry 174

Turkey keema peas 178

Beef stir-fry 180

Lamb dhansak 182

Pork souvlaki with light salsa verde 184

BAKED FISH WITH RED PEPPERS AND TOMATOES

With some good cod, haddock or other fish, this is a breeze to put together and it's so good to eat. It's a great family supper but also just right to serve when friends come over – it's nice to let everyone open their own parcels at the table and enjoy the wafts of delicious saffrony, basily aromas. And it's so low in calories that you can enjoy a few steamed new potatoes and green beans alongside.

200 calories per serving
Serves 4

---

1 tsp olive oil

1 red onion, thinly sliced into wedges

2 red peppers, deseeded and sliced lengthways into strips

2 garlic cloves, finely chopped

1 mild red chilli, deseeded and finely chopped

100ml white wine

pinch of saffron threads

200g canned tomatoes (or fresh)

2 tbsp finely chopped parsley

2 tbsp finely chopped basil

1 tsp grated lemon zest

low-cal olive oil spray

4 thick white fish fillets, about 150g each

4 thin slices of lemon

freshly ground black pepper

Preheat the oven to 200°C/Fan 180°C/Gas 6. Heat the oil in a large non-stick frying pan. Add the onion and red peppers and fry them over a medium heat until they start to soften – you want them to stay fairly firm. Add the garlic and chilli and cook for another 2 minutes, stirring regularly.

Pour the white wine into the pan and crumble in the pinch of saffron. Simmer until most of the wine has evaporated, then add the tomatoes. Cook over a low heat for another 5 minutes, then stir in the parsley, basil and lemon zest.

Cut 4 large pieces of baking paper or foil – they need to be big enough to make a parcel for each fish fillet. Spritz each piece lightly with oil and place a fish fillet in the middle. Season with pepper, then put a thin slice of lemon on top and add a quarter of the red pepper and tomato mixture to each parcel. Bring 2 opposite edges of the paper or foil together and fold them together. Fold over the remaining 2 edges to seal the parcel neatly. Wrap the remaining parcels in the same way.

Place the parcels on a baking tray and put them in the oven. Bake for 12–15 minutes, then open one slightly and check that the fish is cooked through. Take the parcels to the table so that everyone can open their own and enjoy the sensational scents.

WHITE BEAN AND TUNA FISHCAKES

Everyone loves a fishcake, and tuna and white beans are a classic combination. You can use any kind of canned fish you like for this recipe though – such as salmon, sardines or mackerel – as long as it's packed in spring water, as this reduces the calorie count by a lot. BTW, you might be tempted to throw everything into the food processor at once, but take our advice and don't. We've tried making these fishcakes in different ways and it really is worth blitzing the beans and the fish separately to get the right texture – otherwise the beans get too smooth and claggy. And you don't need to wash the food processor in between, so it doesn't take much longer.

175 calories per fishcake
Makes 8 fishcakes

---

2 x 400g cans of cannellini beans, drained and rinsed
2 cans of fish in spring water (drained weight 200–250g)
1 onion, very finely chopped
small bunch of parsley, roughly chopped
2 tsp Dijon mustard
1 egg, beaten
grated zest and juice of 1 lemon

100g wholemeal breadcrumbs
low-cal olive oil spray
freshly ground black pepper

SAUCE (OPTIONAL)
grated zest and juice of 1 lemon
1 tbsp finely chopped capers
1 tbsp finely chopped cornichons
1 tbsp Dijon mustard
150ml 0%-fat yoghurt

Preheat the oven to 220°C/Fan 200°C/Gas 7. Put the
cannellini beans in a food processor and pulse a few times
until they have broken down a little but are not completely
puréed. You want a fairly coarse but uniform texture. Tip the
beans into a large bowl.

Put the drained fish in the food processor with the onion
and parsley and blitz until everything is well combined and
the parsley is very finely chopped. Add this mixture to the
beans in the bowl.

Add the mustard, beaten egg, lemon zest and juice to the
beans and fish, and season with pepper. Mix thoroughly, then
taste again for seasoning and add a little more mustard or
lemon juice if you like.

CONTINUED ON NEXT PAGE

Sprinkle the breadcrumbs over a plate. Shape the fish and bean mixture into 8 patties, dip them in the breadcrumbs, then pat off any excess. Spritz a non-stick baking tray with low-cal oil and place the fishcakes on it. Spritz the top of the fishcakes with oil. Bake the fishcakes in the oven for about 15 minutes, turning them halfway through the cooking time.

While the fishcakes are baking, make the sauce, if using. Simply mix all the ingredients in a bowl and stir well, then season with black pepper. Serve with the fishcakes.

BIKER TIP

If you have time, it is a good idea to chill the mixture in the fridge for a while. It will firm up and be much easier to shape into fishcakes.

Canned fish is a great thing to have in your store cupboard and it contains plenty of protein and nutrients.

MEDITERRANEAN
FISH CASSEROLE

Cooking fish in an aromatic broth in this way is so easy – you can't go wrong. The dish has a really lovely fresh, zingy flavour and brings a touch of Mediterranean sunshine to your table. It's awesomely low in calories too, so you can afford to serve plenty of extra veg alongside. (*See photo on colour plate K.*)

239 calories per serving
Serves 4

---

2 tsp olive oil

1 large fennel bulb, trimmed and sliced into 8 wedges

1 red pepper, cut into strips

300g baby new potatoes, halved if large

2 garlic cloves, finely chopped

1 strip of pared orange zest

1 thyme sprig

150ml white wine

400ml fish or vegetable stock

200g fresh tomatoes, peeled and chopped (or canned equivalent)

4 x 150g white fish fillets, skinned and left whole

freshly ground black pepper

Heat the olive oil in a large flameproof casserole dish. Add the fennel wedges and sear them on both sides until nicely caramelised. Add the red pepper, potatoes and garlic and cook for 3–4 minutes.

Add the orange zest, thyme, white wine and stock. Season with pepper, then bring everything to the boil. Turn down the heat, cover the dish with a lid and leave to simmer for about 10 minutes. Add the tomatoes and continue to cook for another 10 minutes or until the vegetables are tender.

Season the fish fillets with pepper, then place them on top of the vegetables. Cover the dish and leave the fish to steam for 7–8 minutes. Serve in wide, shallow bowls.

FISH CURRY

A hot and sour curry, this has a lovely fresh taste and is very simple to make. What's more, it's nice and low in calories so you can treat yourself to a chapati as well if you fancy. If you're a curry fan you'll probably have some tamarind paste in your larder, but if not it's available in most supermarkets and it does add a good tangy flavour. (*See photo on colour plate K.*)

226 calories per serving
Serves 4

---

1 tbsp vegetable oil

2 onions, thinly sliced

3 garlic cloves, finely chopped

10g chunk of fresh root ginger, finely chopped

4 medium tomatoes or 400g canned chopped tomatoes

1 tbsp Kashmiri chilli powder or 2 tsp sweet paprika and
  1 tsp cayenne

2 tsp ground cumin

1 tsp ground coriander

½ tsp turmeric

300ml hot fish stock or water

2 tbsp tamarind paste

juice of 1 lime

600g skinned firm white fish fillets (hake or tilapia)

handful of chopped coriander
freshly ground black pepper

Heat the oil in a large shallow pan. You need one that has a lid and is wide enough to take all the fish in one layer. Add the onions and stir to coat them with the oil. Cover the pan and leave the onions over a low heat for 5 minutes to start softening while you prepare the garlic and ginger.

If using fresh tomatoes, remove the cores, then blitz them in a blender and set them aside.

Add the garlic and ginger to the onions and cook for a further minute. Sprinkle the spices into the pan and stir briefly to combine. Add the hot fish stock or water and season with pepper. Simmer for 5 minutes, then add the tomatoes and tamarind paste. Bring the curry to the boil, then turn down the heat and leave to cook uncovered for another 5 minutes, then add some of the lime juice. Taste the curry, then add more lime juice if you like, but don't overdo it. You don't want the curry to taste too sour.

Cut the fish into large chunks and sit these on top of the sauce, pressing them down very lightly. Cover the pan and cook for 3–4 minutes or until the fish is cooked through. Sprinkle with chopped coriander and serve at once.

SALMON AND BROCCOLI TRAY BAKE

The beauty of a tray bake is that all the flavours work together and you get lots of lovely little caramelised bits to enjoy. The honey and vinegar add little touches of sweetness and tartness, which go perfectly with the salmon. This dish is higher in calories than some in this book, but it is a well balanced and nutritious meal. (*See photo on colour plate N.*)

446 calories per serving
Serves 4

½ tsp honey

2 tsp balsamic vinegar

1 garlic clove, crushed

4 x 150g salmon fillets, skinned

1 large head of broccoli, broken into florets

200g baby salad potatoes, halved lengthways

1 red pepper, thickly sliced

1 red onion, sliced into thin wedges

low-cal olive oil spray

250g white cup mushrooms, left whole

small bunch of basil leaves

freshly ground black pepper

Preheat the oven to 200°C/Fan 180°C/Gas 6. To make the marinade for the salmon, mix the honey, balsamic vinegar and garlic in a bowl and season with pepper. Brush this mixture over both sides of the salmon and leave it to marinate while you start cooking the vegetables.

Wash the broccoli and, without brushing off too much of the water, put it in a roasting tin. Add the potatoes, red pepper and onion, then spritz with some oil. Roast the vegetables in the oven for 20 minutes.

Add the salmon and mushrooms to the tin and roast for another 12 minutes until the salmon is just cooked through. Remove the tin from the oven and add a few basil leaves, then serve the tray bake immediately.

MACKEREL FILLETS WITH GREMOLATA

Gremolata is the name for a simple but tasty Italian garnish. It's just finely chopped garlic, parsley and lemon zest but it adds a fantastic zingy flavour to chicken, meat or fish, such as this super-speedy mackerel dish. We've suggested cooking the fish in a frying pan with just a light spritz of oil, but you could also grill it on a griddle or a barbecue if you like – using one of those handy fish cages. This is lovely served with a tomato and onion salad. (*See photo on colour plate M.*)

339 calories per serving
Serves 2

---

4 small mackerel fillets, about 300g in total
low-cal olive oil spray
2 tbsp finely chopped flatleaf parsley
2 garlic cloves, finely chopped
finely grated zest of 1 lemon
freshly ground black pepper

TOMATO AND ONION SALAD
1 small sweet white onion, finely sliced into crescents
2 or 3 very ripe vine tomatoes

1 tsp olive oil

squeeze of lemon juice

1 tbsp finely chopped flatleaf parsley

1 tsp capers (optional)

finely ground white pepper

First check your mackerel fillets for pin bones – those pesky little bones left behind when the fish is filleted. Remove as many as you can with a pair of tweezers – makes the fish even nicer to eat.

Lightly spray a large non-stick frying pan with oil and place it over a medium heat. Season the mackerel fillets with black pepper. Put the fillets in the pan, skin-side down, and cook for 3–4 minutes. When the flesh of the mackerel is almost completely white and opaque, turn the fillets over and cook for another minute.

Mix the parsley, garlic and lemon zest together to make the gremolata. Serve the mackerel with the gremolata on the side, for sprinkling over.

CONTINUED ON NEXT PAGE

Tomato and onion salad

Soaking onions before using them raw takes off that really astringent edge. But if you don't mind that, you can leave out the soaking step.

Put the onion slices in a bowl of very cold water. Leave them for 10 minutes, then drain. Slice the tomatoes horizontally into thin rounds and arrange them on a plate. Sprinkle over the onion crescents.

Whisk together the olive oil, lemon juice and white pepper. Pour this over the tomatoes and onions. Sprinkle over the parsley and the capers, if using. Leave for a few minutes to allow the flavours to develop, then serve at room temperature.

Fish is an excellent
choice if you
are trying to
lose weight, and
although oily
fish is higher in
calories than white
fish, it's good
for heart health
so is still highly
recommended.

FISH CRUMBLE

The only thing that's humble about this crumble is the calorie count! Cod, haddock or hake all work well and the smoked fish adds a nice touch of extra flavour. The creamy sauce contrasts brilliantly with the crunchy couscous topping, which we reckon is genius and much lower in calories than mashed potato. We like to use wholewheat couscous for the extra fibre. This dish is healthy, delicious and an easy way to cook fish. We reckon you're going to love it. (*See photo on colour plate N.*)

388 calories per serving
Serves 4

600g skinless white fish fillets, cut into chunks
150g smoked haddock fillets, cut into chunks
low-cal olive oil spray
white pepper

SAUCE
1 slice of onion
2 bay leaves
a few white peppercorns
50ml white wine
50ml semi-skimmed milk
200ml reduced-fat crème fraiche

1 tsp plain flour
25g reduced-fat extra-mature Cheddar cheese
small bunch of parsley

COUSCOUS TOPPING
100g wholewheat couscous
120ml just-boiled water
25g reduced-fat, extra-mature Cheddar cheese
2 tsp olive oil

Preheat the oven to 200°C/Fan 180°C/Gas 6. To prepare the couscous, tip it into a heatproof bowl and pour over the just-boiled water. Cover and leave the couscous to stand until all the water has been absorbed, then fluff it up with a fork.

For the sauce, put the onion and bay leaves in a saucepan with the peppercorns. Pour in the wine and milk, then stir in the crème fraiche. Put the pan over a low heat and whisk in the flour and cheese.

When the sauce is well combined and the cheese has melted, leave to simmer gently for a couple of minutes, then add the white fish and the smoked haddock. Continue to simmer for 3–4 minutes until the fish is just cooked through, then remove from the heat.

CONTINUED ON NEXT PAGE

Finely chop the parsley and set aside 2 tablespoons. Stir the rest into the sauce. Spritz a shallow ovenproof dish with oil. Spoon the fish and sauce into the dish and season with some white pepper.

Now add the topping. Mix the reserved chopped parsley with the couscous and spoon it over the sauce. Sprinkle the cheese on top – it will stop the couscous from crisping up too much – then drizzle over the olive oil.

Bake the crumble in the preheated oven for about 10 minutes until everything is piping hot. Serve with lots of lovely seasonal green vegetables.

If you feel like second helpings, wait 20 minutes. It takes about that time for the message that you're full to get to your brain – and you'll probably find that you don't need more food after all.

CHILLI PRAWN PASTA

With chilli, garlic and lime, this pasta dish is brimming with bold flavours and makes a proper filling dinner. If you do happen to have some vodka handy, we recommend adding a dash. It brings a touch of extra magic to the dish. (*See photo on colour plate N.*)

341 calories per serving
Serves 4

200g wholewheat spaghetti

1 small onion, finely chopped

1 red pepper, deseeded and finely chopped

2 garlic cloves, finely chopped

1 tbsp olive oil

1 tsp chilli flakes

grated zest of 1 lime

100ml hot fish or vegetable stock

250ml tomato passata

50ml vodka (optional)

400g shelled raw prawns (defrosted if frozen)

small bunch of coriander or basil, to garnish

lime wedges, to serve

freshly ground black pepper

Bring a pan of water to the boil and cook the pasta until it is tender but still with a little bite to it, then drain.

Heat the olive oil in a large lidded frying pan, then add the onion and red pepper along with a splash of water. Cover the pan and cook over a medium heat until the veg are starting to soften. Add the garlic, chilli flakes and lime zest, then season with pepper. Pour the stock into the pan, put the lid back on and cook the sauce for another 5 minutes.

Pour in the passata and simmer for a further 5 minutes.
Add the vodka, if using, then simmer for a minute or so more.
Throw in the prawns and cook until they have just turned pink and opaque – they should still be quite bouncy.

Serve the sauce with the pasta and a sprinkling of coriander or basil leaves to garnish. Add some lime wedges for everyone to squeeze over their helping.

TURKEY CHILLI WITH CAULIFLOWER 'RICE'

You can add a tiny bit of chocolate to this chilli which gives it a lovely rich mouth feel, but don't be tempted to eat the rest of the bar! Instead of serving the chilli with regular rice, try our cauliflower version, which tastes great and is very low calorie. Chipotle paste is available in supermarkets and delivers a real kick to the dish. (*See photo on colour plate M.*)

300 calories per serving (with cauliflower)
240 calories (without cauliflower)
Serves 4

---

1 tsp vegetable oil

1 red onion, finely chopped

1 large red pepper, deseeded and diced

2 celery sticks, trimmed and diced

4 garlic cloves, finely chopped

500g turkey mince

1 tsp dried oregano

2 bay leaves

1 tbsp ground cumin

½ tsp ground allspice

1 tbsp chipotle paste

400g can of chopped tomatoes
400g can of beans (kidney, black-eyed beans), drained and
   rinsed
15g dark chocolate
freshly ground black pepper

To serve
fresh coriander leaves
lime wedges, for squeezing
reduced-fat crème fraiche

CAULIFLOWER RICE
1 cauliflower, broken up into florets
1 tsp cumin seeds
small bunch of fresh coriander, chopped

Heat the oil in a large saucepan, then add the onion, pepper
and celery. Cook over a low heat for 5 minutes, until the veg
are starting to soften, then add the garlic and the turkey
mince. Turn up the heat slightly and cook until the turkey has
browned all over. Keep stirring and use the spoon to break up
any clumps of turkey mince.

Add the oregano, bay leaves, cumin, allspice and chipotle
paste. Give everything a good stir so it all gets coated with the
paste, then pour in the chopped tomatoes and 250ml of water.

CONTINUED ON NEXT PAGE

Add the drained beans and season with black pepper. Bring to the boil, then cover the pan and simmer the chilli over a low heat for half an hour, until the sauce has thickened. Keep an eye on it and add a drop more water towards the end if you think it is in danger of catching.

Five minutes from the end of the cooking time, add the chocolate. To serve, divide between 4 plates, sprinkle with coriander leaves and add a wedge of lime and a dessertspoon of crème fraiche to each serving.

Cauliflower rice

Put the cauliflower florets in a food processor and blitz until the cauliflower has the texture of large breadcrumbs.

Heat a non-stick frying pan and dry-fry the cumin seeds for a few moments until they start to give off a spicy aroma. Coat the bottom of the pan with water – about 100ml should do it. Evenly spread the cauliflower crumbs over the frying pan and season with pepper. Cook over a medium heat for about 5 minutes, stirring fairly regularly until the water has evaporated and the cauliflower is looking quite dry.

Stir in the coriander and remove the pan from the heat. Fork the cauliflower over and it will 'fluff up' nicely. Serve with the turkey chilli.

Cauliflower is a great low-cal side dish. There's only 25 calories in 100 grams so you can eat plenty of it!

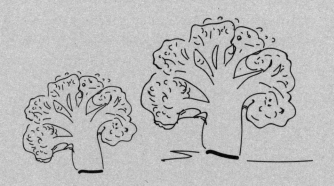

GARLIC CHICKEN WITH BEANS, KALE AND CHERRY TOMATOES

Slicing chicken breasts in half like this creates two nice thin pieces from each breast. This way they cook quickly without getting tough. The rest is easy and makes a good simple meal.

290 calories per serving
Serves 4

---

4 chicken breasts, skinned

1 tbsp olive oil

4 garlic cloves, crushed

200g kale, shredded

400g can of cannellini beans, drained and rinsed

300g cherry tomatoes, halved

1 tbsp sherry vinegar

freshly ground black pepper

UNDER 270 CALORIES

1.

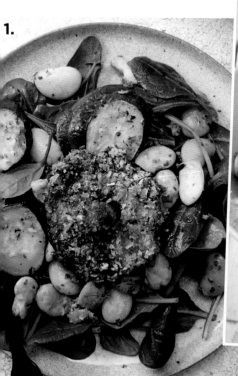

2.

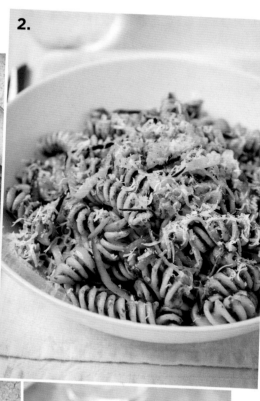

3.

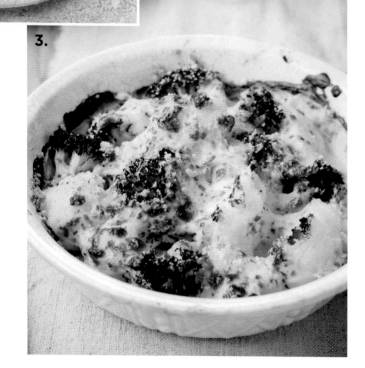

1. Pesto-stuffed
   mushrooms
   (209 cals, p.128)

2. Green pasta
   (239 cals, p.120)

3. Cauliflower and
   broccoli cheese
   (261 cals, p.126)

VEGGIE TREATS

UNDER 350 CALORIES

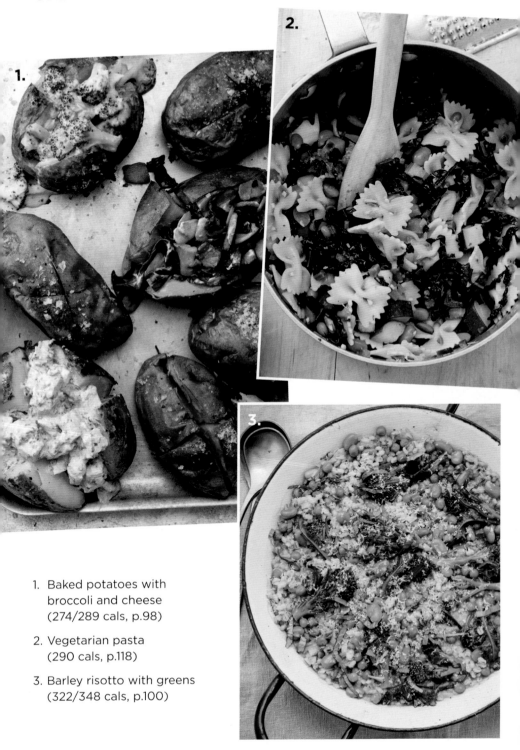

1. Baked potatoes with broccoli and cheese (274/289 cals, p.98)

2. Vegetarian pasta (290 cals, p.118)

3. Barley risotto with greens (322/348 cals, p.100)

UNDER 270 CALORIES

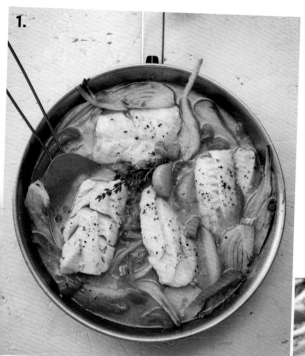

1 Mediterranean fish casserole (239 cals, p.148)

2. Fish curry (226 cals, p.150)

3. Pork souvlaki with light salsa verde (270/180 cals, p.184)

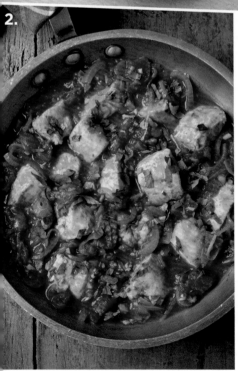

HEARTY SUPPERS

UNDER 300 CALORIES

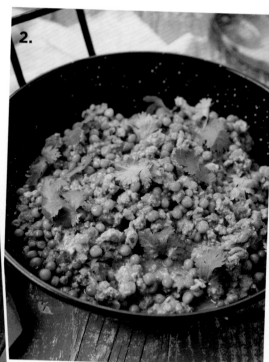

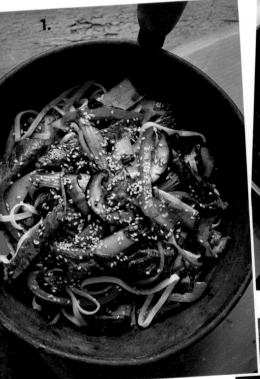

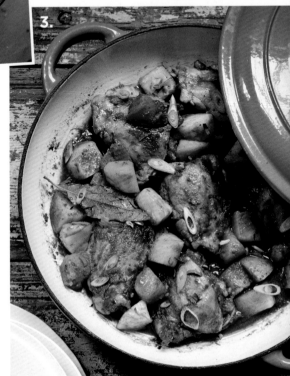

1. Beef stir-fry
   (283 cals, p.180)

2. Turkey keema peas
   (270 cals, p.178)

3. Caribbean chicken curry
   (290 cals, p.174)

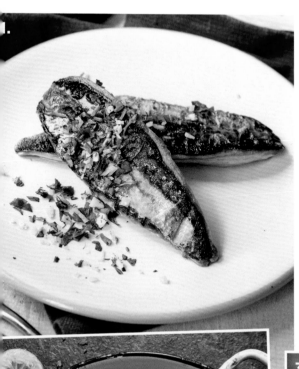

1. Mackerel fillets with gremolata
   (339 cals, p.154)

2. Lamb dhansak
   (336 cals, p.182)

3. Turkey chilli with cauliflower 'rice'
   (300 cals, p.164)

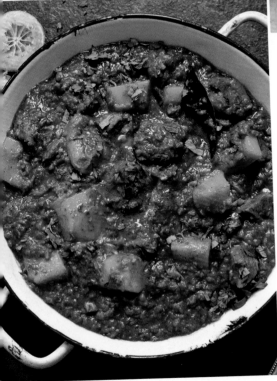

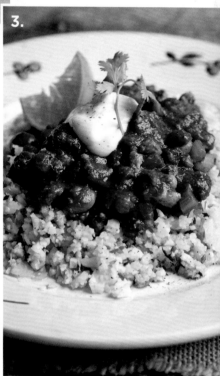

HEARTY SUPPERS

UNDER 450 CALORIES

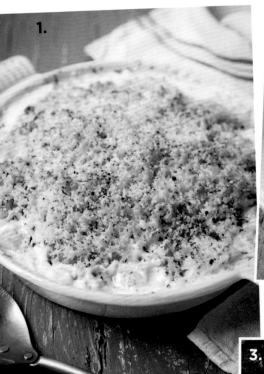

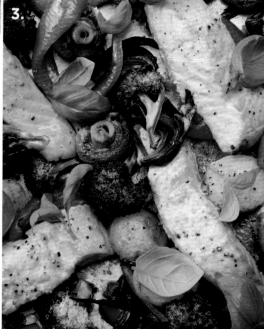

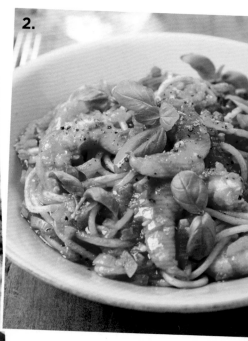

1 Fish crumble
   (388 cals, p.158)

2. Chilli prawn pasta
   (341 cals, p.162)

3. Salmon and broccoli tray
   bake (446 cals, p.152)

UNDER 200 CALORIES

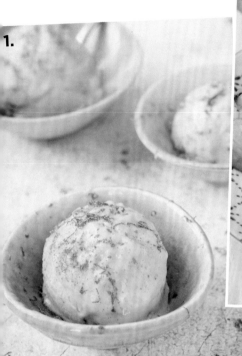

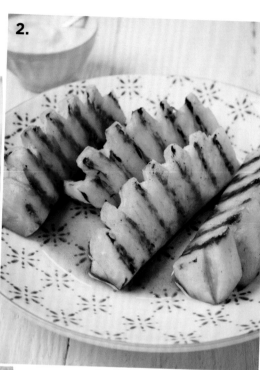

1. Instant banana ice cream
(100/67 cals, p.224)

2. Grilled pineapple
(92 cals, p.226)

3. Crunchy oat cookies
(156 cals each, p.240)

PUDDINGS AND BAKES

UNDER 220 CALORIES

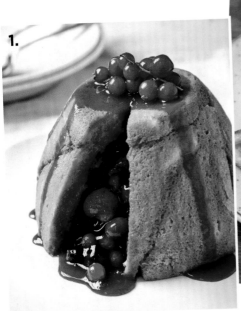

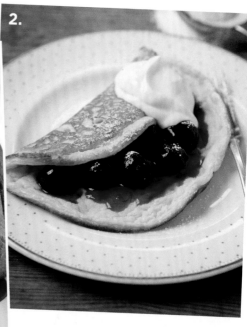

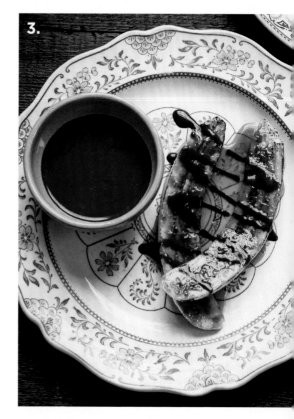

1. Summer pudding
   (131 cals, p.218)

2. Sweet omelette
   (217 cals, p.228)

3. Baked bananas with
   chocolate rum sauce
   (194 cals, p.234)

First prepare the chicken. Place each breast on a work surface with the top side facing up. Put one hand on the chicken breast, then slice through into the side of the breast, continuing to slice horizontally until you have cut all the way through.

Put the olive oil and crushed garlic in a bowl. Season the chicken pieces well with black pepper, then add them to the bowl. Rub the chicken breasts with the garlicky oil until they are all thoroughly coated, then if you have time, leave them to marinate for half an hour.

When you are ready to cook the chicken, heat a large griddle pan until it is too hot to hold your hand over, then turn the heat down to medium. Cook the chicken breasts for 3–4 minutes on each side until they have char lines and are completely cooked through. You may need to do this in a couple of batches. If so, keep the first batch warm while you cook the second batch.

Meanwhile, bring a large pan of water to the boil. Cook the kale for 3 minutes until almost done, then add the beans to heat through for a minute. Drain well.

To assemble, divide the kale and beans between 4 plates. Cut the chicken breasts diagonally into strips and add them to the plates. Sprinkle over the cherry tomatoes, then drizzle over the sherry vinegar and serve immediately.

FUSION TANDOORI CHICKEN

We originally created this bit of fusion confusion for salmon but tried it with chicken and it was even better. You'll think that mixing tandoori paste, dill and capers sounds like a crazy idea but trust us, it really works! Great with some brown rice and salad alongside.

214 calories per serving (2 drumsticks)
321 calories per serving (3 drumsticks)
Serves 4–6

---

12 chicken drumsticks, skinned

100g low-fat natural yoghurt

2 tbsp chopped dill

2 tbsp capers

100g tandoori paste

1 tsp chilli powder (optional)

lemon wedges, to serve

Cut slashes in the flesh of the drumsticks, then put them in a bowl. Put the yoghurt, dill and capers in a blender or food processor and blitz until the capers and dill are finely chopped. Mix this with the tandoori paste, and the chilli powder if you want some extra heat, then pour the lot over the chicken.

Make sure the paste covers the chicken – the best way to do this is to massage it into the cuts with your hands. Cover and leave to marinate for at least an hour, but preferably overnight.

When you're ready to cook the chicken, preheat the oven to its highest setting. Put a wire rack over a roasting tin. Take the drumsticks out of the marinade and place them on the rack. Bake for 20–25 minutes, turning occasionally, until the drumsticks are well cooked and starting to blacken in places. Serve with lemon wedges to squeeze over the chicken.

CHICKEN TRAY BAKE WITH FENNEL, PEAS AND NEW POTATOES

A chicken tray bake is a trusty favourite for both of us and we're really pleased with this version. We reckon it will be a go-to supper in households around the country. There are lots of lovely flavours and a good range of textures, thanks to all the different vegetables.

343 calories per serving
Serves 4

---

1 large or 2 small fennel bulbs, trimmed and sliced into
   8 wedges
200g baby new potatoes, sliced lengthways
8 skinless, boneless chicken thigh fillets, trimmed of any fat
100ml white wine
juice and zest of 1 lemon
1 tsp dried thyme
300g peas
2 little gem lettuces, halved lengthways
low-cal olive oil spray
freshly ground black pepper

Preheat the oven to 200°C/Fan 180°C/Gas 6. Arrange the fennel and potatoes in a large roasting tin, then drape the chicken thighs on top, partially covering the fennel. Pour over the white wine and lemon juice, then sprinkle on the zest and thyme. Season generously with pepper.

Cover the tin with foil and put it in the oven for 30 minutes. Then remove the tin from the oven, take off the foil and pour the peas in around the chicken. Uncover the fennel and potatoes as you go – you want them to crisp up, not to be smothered in peas. Tuck in the little gems around the veg.

Spritz with oil, then bake for another 30–35 minutes, uncovered, until the potatoes and fennel are tender and the potatoes have crisped up a bit around the edges.

CARIBBEAN CHICKEN CURRY

This is a proper carnival of a dish and has everything you need in one scrumptious pot full of Caribbean flavours. You can buy Caribbean curry powder in most supermarkets or make your own – see our tip on page 176. (*See photo on colour plate L.*)

290 calories per serving
Serves 4

---

8 bone-in chicken thighs, skinned and trimmed of fat

1½ limes

1 tbsp vegetable oil

300ml chicken stock or water

1 large thyme sprig

2 bay leaves

200g piece of pumpkin, peeled and cut into large chunks

1 large potato, peeled and cut into large chunks

100g pineapple, diced

1 tsp rum (optional)

2 spring onions, finely sliced

2 tbsp chopped flatleaf parsley

freshly ground black pepper

CURRY PASTE

1 onion, roughly chopped

4 garlic cloves, peeled and halved

15g chunk of fresh root ginger, peeled and roughly chopped

2 scotch bonnet chillies (or to taste), deseeded and finely
   chopped

2 tbsp medium curry powder, preferably Caribbean

½ tsp ground allspice

Put the chicken thighs in a bowl and add the juice of 1 lime and
about 100ml of water. Rub the lime juice over the chicken and
leave for a few minutes while you make the paste.

For the paste, put the onion, garlic, ginger, scotch bonnets,
curry powder and ground allspice in a food processor or
blender and add a tablespoon of water. Blitz until the mixture
is fairly smooth.

Heat the vegetable oil in a large flameproof casserole
dish over a medium heat. Add the paste and cook, stirring
constantly, for a couple of minutes. Now add the chicken and
season with pepper. Stir so the chicken is coated with the
paste, then pour in 300ml of chicken stock or water and add
the thyme and bay leaves.

Bring the mixture to the boil, then turn down the heat to a
gentle simmer and cover. Cook for about 45 minutes, before

CONTINUED ON NEXT PAGE

adding the pumpkin, potato and pineapple. Cook for another 30 minutes, covered, then take off the lid. Add the juice of the remaining half a lime and, if you like, a teaspoon of rum, then cook, uncovered, for another 10 minutes to allow the sauce to reduce a little. Sprinkle the spring onions and parsley over the top of the curry and serve.

BIKER TIP _____

If you fancy making your own Caribbean curry powder, dry fry a 4cm piece of cinnamon stick, broken up, with 2 tablespoons of coriander seeds, 2 teaspoons of cumin seeds, 1 teaspoon of mustard seeds, 1 teaspoon of white peppercorns, half a teaspoon of allspice berries, half a teaspoon of fenugreek, seeds from 6 cardamom pods, 4 cloves, 2 mace blades and 2 dried bay leaves in a dry frying pan. Toast until their aroma intensifies and the mustard seeds start popping. Transfer to a bowl to cool.

Grind the spices in a spice grinder or with a pestle and mortar, then mix with a tablespoon of turmeric and half a teaspoon of onion salt. Store in an airtight jar.

Spices and spice mixes are great for bringing your cooking alive and adding bags of flavour but few calories.

TURKEY KEEMA PEAS

The trad keema pea dish is made with lamb, but our turkey mince version has far fewer calories and still tastes awesome. Best to get minced turkey thigh, rather than breast which will dry out more, or if you have a friendly local butcher, you could ask for minced chicken thighs, which will also work well. (*See photo on colour plate L.*)

270 calories per serving
Serves 4

---

1 tsp vegetable oil

1 onion, finely chopped

2 garlic cloves, finely chopped

10g chunk of fresh root ginger, grated

small bunch of coriander, stems and leaves separated, stems finely chopped

1 tbsp mild curry powder

600g turkey thigh mince

1 bay leaf

400g can of chopped tomatoes

200ml reduced-fat coconut milk

250g petits pois, defrosted

freshly ground black pepper

Heat the oil in a large lidded saucepan. Add the onion and fry it briskly over a high heat for a couple of minutes, stirring regularly, then add the garlic and ginger. Fry and stir for another minute.

Add the coriander leaves, curry powder and mince. Stir until the mince has browned slightly and is well coated with the spices. Add the bay leaf and pour in the tomatoes and the coconut milk. Season with pepper.

Bring to the boil and cover the pan again. Simmer over a medium heat for 5 minutes, then take the lid off the pan and add the peas. Bring to the boil again, stir thoroughly, then turn down the heat and leave the mixture to simmer, uncovered, for another 10 minutes until the sauce has thickened. Serve sprinkled with plenty of coriander leaves.

A small portion of rice or some cauliflower rice (see page 166) alongside is nice. The cauli rice only adds another 60 calories per portion.

BEEF STIR-FRY

Stir-fries are the dieter's best friend when you want something healthy, filling and fast, and this one completely fills the bill. It's inspired by dishes we ate on our trip to Korea a few years ago. Just keep your portion of noodles down and fill up on all the lovely vegetables. (*See photo on colour plate L.*)

283 calories per serving
Serves 4

100g rice noodles
½ tsp sesame oil
300g steak (sirloin, flank, bavette or rump)
1 tbsp vegetable oil
1 red pepper, deseeded and sliced into strips
1 large carrot, cut into matchsticks
4 spring onions, cut into 1cm rounds
200g shiitake mushrooms
2 garlic cloves, finely chopped
5g chunk of fresh root ginger, finely chopped
large bag of pak choi or other Asian greens
2 tbsp soy sauce (preferably a low-sodium version)
1 tsp rice wine vinegar
1 tsp sesame seeds (white or black), to serve

First cook the noodles, according to the packet instructions, then drain and toss them in the sesame oil. Trim the beef of any fat and cut the meat into thin strips.

Heat the vegetable oil in a wok. Add the red pepper and carrot and stir-fry for 3 minutes over a high heat. Add the spring onions and mushrooms and cook for another 2 minutes, then add the beef, garlic and ginger. Continue to stir-fry until the beef is seared on all sides.

Trim the pak choi or greens and slice them if the leaves are large. Pour the soy sauce and rice wine vinegar into the wok and add the greens, then cook over a slightly lower heat until the greens have wilted down. Add the noodles and warm them through. Serve at once, sprinkled with sesame seeds.

LAMB DHANSAK

This is a proper Friday night curry and we've trimmed the calories while keeping it punchy and delicious. A richly satisfying dish. (*See photo on colour plate M.*)

336 calories per serving
Serves 6

---

1 tbsp vegetable oil

2 large onions, thinly sliced

750g lean lamb leg meat, diced

20g chunk of fresh root ginger, peeled and grated

4 garlic cloves, finely chopped

3 green chillies, deseeded and finely chopped

2 tbsp medium curry powder

1 tbsp ground cumin

1 tbsp ground coriander

1 tsp turmeric

2 bay leaves

150g red lentils

½ butternut squash, cut into large chunks

juice of 1 lime

handful of coriander leaves, chopped, to garnish

freshly ground black pepper

Heat the oil in a large flameproof casserole dish or a heavy-based pan. Add the onions and cook over a low heat until they have softened but not browned. This should take about 15 minutes. Turn up the heat slightly and add the lamb, ginger, garlic and chillies. Sprinkle all the spices over the meat and season with pepper. Stir for a couple of minutes until the lamb is well coated with spices.

Add the bay leaves and the red lentils, then pour in 700ml of water. Slowly bring it to the boil, turn the heat down and leave to simmer for an hour. Add the butternut squash and cook for another half an hour, then remove the lid and leave the curry to simmer, uncovered, for another 15 minutes.

Check the seasoning, add the lime juice and sprinkle with chopped coriander before serving. Lovely served with some rice or cauliflower rice (see page 166).

BIKER TIP

This freezes well. The flavours of the ginger and garlic will intensify on freezing, but in a good way. Just be careful when defrosting and reheating not to stir too much, as cooked, frozen lamb has a tendency to shred. To avoid soggy butternut squash, prepare the dish up to the point before adding the squash, then freeze and add the butternut squash when reheating.

PORK SOUVLAKI WITH LIGHT SALSA VERDE

These pork kebabs are satisfaction on a stick. Salsa verde goes beautifully with them but usually contains shedloads of olive oil. We've come up with something that's more like a herby mayonnaise and we really love it – see what you think. Just so you know – the sauce does contain raw egg. (*See photo on colour plate K.*)

270 **calories per serving (4)**
180 **calories per serving (6)**
Serves 4–6

700g lean pork, diced into 3cm chunks

MARINADE
1 tsp olive oil
juice of 1 lemon
1 tsp dried mint
1 tsp dried oregano
1 bay leaf, crumbled
1 tbsp red wine vinegar
freshly ground black pepper

LIGHT SALSA VERDE

1 egg yolk

1 heaped tsp Dijon mustard

1 tbsp olive oil

juice of 1 lemon

2 anchovies, finely chopped (optional)

2 tbsp capers, rinsed and chopped

large bunch of flatleaf parsley leaves, finely chopped

small bunch of basil, finely chopped

small bunch of mint, finely chopped

freshly ground black pepper

Mix all the marinade ingredients together in a large non-metallic bowl. Add the chunks of pork and stir until they are all completely covered, then leave the meat to marinate in the fridge for at least half an hour. It's fine to leave it overnight if you have the time.

For the light salsa verde, put the egg yolk in a bowl with the mustard. Whisk them together, then add the olive oil, a few drops at a time, so the mixture emulsifies properly. Whisk in the lemon juice, then stir in all the remaining ingredients. If you want a very smooth sauce, blitz it briefly in a blender. You can also add a tablespoon of water if you prefer the sauce to be slightly thinner.

CONTINUED ON NEXT PAGE

If you're using bamboo skewers, soak them in water for half an hour before you need them – this will prevent them from burning. Thread the pork chunks on to 8 skewers. Cook the souvlaki on a hot barbecue, on a griddle pan on the hob (you may have to do this in batches) or under a hot grill, for 12–15 minutes. Turn the skewers regularly, until all the meat is charred and cooked through.

Serve the pork kebabs on or off the skewers, with the sauce on the side and a simple salad.

It really does help to take your time over meals. Eat slowly, chew your food well and put your fork down in between every mouthful. You'll find you enjoy everything more – and you'll eat less.

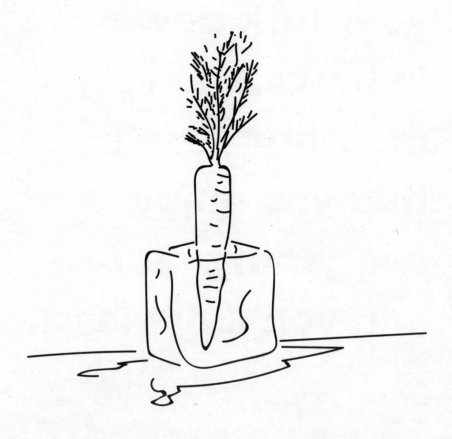

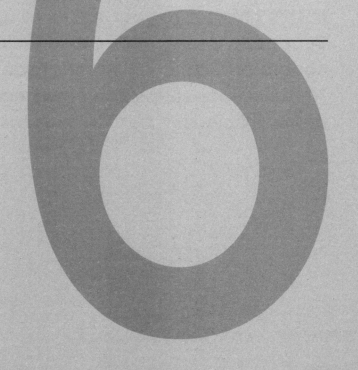

SIDES
and
BASICS

6

As we all know, vegetables are our best friends when we want to lose weight and stay healthy. They provide plenty of vitamins and nutrients and also really help to fill you up and keep you satisfied. What's more, most veg are low in calories so you can eat loads of them without breaking your calorie budget. Make sure you have at least five portions of veg a day and your body will thank you for it. Try adding some of the dishes in this chapter to your meals to up your vegetable intake. We've also included a couple of recipes for home-made stocks to make your soups and stews even more delicious.

Roast spiced cauliflower 192

Red cabbage with apple and chestnuts 194

Root vegetable boulangère 196

Spring greens with harissa and garlic 198

Root vegetable rösti 200

Greek-style roast vegetables 202

Rainbow vegetable 'couscous' 204

Home-made baked beans 206

Tomato sauce 208

Vegetable stock 210

Chicken stock 212

ROAST SPICED CAULIFLOWER

Serve this with curries, casseroles or any other dish you would usually eat with rice. You'll find it soaks up juices beautifully without loading you with calories.

25 calories per serving
Serves 4

½ head of cauliflower, broken into florets

1 tsp vegetable oil

1 tsp nigella seeds (optional)

1 tsp cumin seeds

1 tsp coriander seeds

1 tsp mustard seeds (optional)

grated zest and juice of 1 lime

freshly ground black pepper

Preheat the oven to 200°C/Fan 180°C/Gas 6. Bring a large pan of water to the boil and add the cauliflower florets. Cook for 2 minutes, then drain and leave to dry out in the colander.

Give the seeds a light pounding with a pestle and mortar or bash them with a rolling pin. Put the cauliflower in a roasting dish and toss with the vegetable oil. Sprinkle over the spices and the lime zest and juice, then season. Roast in the oven for about 15 minutes, until the cauliflower has started to brown round the edges. It should still be slightly firm.

RED CABBAGE WITH APPLE AND CHESTNUTS

Many red cabbage recipes need a long cooking time and contain quite a bit of sugar. We've cut down on both here and the result is quick and delicious – and the cabbage keeps its colour. The recipe does make quite a large quantity but freezes brilliantly, so stash some away for another meal if you don't need it all.

76 calories per serving
Serves 8

---

1 tbsp vegetable oil

1 onion, finely chopped

2 garlic cloves, finely chopped

2 eating apples, peeled and grated or finely chopped

1 small red cabbage, quartered, cored and shredded

a pinch of cinnamon

½ tsp allspice

1 tsp brown sugar (optional)

100g vacuum-packed chestnuts, roughly chopped

1 tbsp cider vinegar

freshly ground black pepper

Heat the oil in a large saucepan. Add the onion and cook for a few minutes until soft, then add the garlic and cook for another 2 minutes.

Now add the apples and cabbage, season with pepper, then sprinkle over the cinnamon, allspice and sugar. Add the chestnuts. Stir the cider vinegar into 100ml of water and pour this into the pan.

Cover and simmer for about 20 minutes until the red cabbage has softened slightly but still has its deep colour.

ROOT VEGETABLE BOULANGÈRE

A lovely comforting dish, this was traditionally made just with potatoes. Our version replaces some of the potato with parsnips and carrots to keep the calories down and give extra flavour. It's good on its own or goes well with grilled meat.

127 calories per serving (4)
85 calories per serving (6)
Serves 4-6

---

1 large or 2 small parsnips (about 300g peeled weight)

2 large carrots (about 250g peeled weight)

2 large potatoes, King Edwards are good (about 400g peeled weight)

low-cal olive oil spray

1 tsp dried sage

2 garlic cloves, finely chopped

600ml vegetable or chicken stock

freshly ground black pepper

Preheat the oven to 200°C/Fan 180°C/Gas 6.

Prepare the vegetables. If the parsnips are fat enough, cut them into rounds, otherwise slice into lengths, as thinly as possible. The carrots should also be sliced thinly, but on the diagonal. Finally, cut the potatoes into slightly thicker slices – about 2–3mm thick.

Spritz a baking dish lightly with oil. Arrange the parsnips over the base – you should have enough for at least 2 layers, perhaps 3 if you have managed to slice them very thinly. Follow with half the sage and garlic, then season lightly with black pepper.

Add a layer of carrots, then repeat the sage, garlic and seasoning. Finally, top with the potatoes.

Make up the stock with boiling water, or heat gently if using fresh stock, and pour this over the vegetables. Cover the baking dish with a single layer of foil and bake in the preheated oven for half an hour. Uncover the baking dish and cook for another half an hour or until the vegetables are tender and most of the liquid has evaporated.

SPRING GREENS WITH HARISSA AND GARLIC

Make this as hot or not as you like. A teaspoon of harissa paste, available in most supermarkets, gives a mellow heat while a tablespoon packs more of a punch – up to you.

41 calories per serving
Serves 4

---

1 tsp olive oil

2 garlic cloves, finely chopped

1 tsp–1 tbsp harissa paste, to taste

400g bag of spring greens, washed and finely shredded

freshly grated zest of 1 lemon

freshly ground black pepper

Heat the olive oil in a large frying pan or saucepan with a lid. Add the garlic cloves and harissa paste and cook for a couple of minutes, stirring constantly.

Add 100ml of water and stir to combine with the garlic and paste, then add the greens. Turn the greens over so they are coated with the sauce, then season with pepper.

Cover and cook over a medium heat for about 5 minutes, stirring every so often, until the spring greens have wilted, but still have a little bite to them. Add the lemon zest at the last minute, just before serving.

ROOT VEGETABLE RÖSTI

Like the boulangère on page 196, this is usually made with potatoes but we like to use a variety of veg. A great way to enjoy some of your five a day.

239 calories per serving (4)
160 calories per serving (6)
Serves 4–6

---

1 parsnip, coarsely grated

1 medium potato, coarsely grated

1 medium beetroot, coarsely grated

1 sweet potato, coarsely grated

200g celeriac, coarsely grated

1 eating apple, coarsely grated

1 small onion, finely chopped

1 tsp chopped sage (optional)

25g plain flour

1 egg

low-cal olive oil spray

1 tbsp olive oil (optional)

freshly ground black pepper

Preheat the oven to 200°C/Fan 180°C/Gas 6.

Bring a large pan of water to the boil and add the grated parsnip, potato, beetroot, sweet potato and celeriac. Boil them for just 2 minutes, then drain them thoroughly and tip them into a bowl. Add the apple and onion to the bowl, then season with pepper. Sprinkle in the sage, if using, and the flour, then mix in the egg.

Spritz a baking tray with low-cal oil. Arrange the vegetable mixture on the baking tray to make a circle measuring about 20cm in diameter.

If you have a loose-bottomed cake tin of this size, you could use it for guidance.

Press the mixture down, making sure it is spread evenly. Drizzle with the tablespoon of olive oil, if using, otherwise spray the rösti again with low-cal oil.

Bake the rösti in the oven for about 40 minutes until it's tender in the middle and crisp and well browned on the outside.

GREEK-STYLE ROAST VEGETABLES

This kind of one-pot vegetable dish usually contains loads of olive oil and so is high in calories. We've found that you can get away with just a small amount of oil and loads of juicy veg and it still tastes fantastic. The veg are good cold too, so make extra and add them to a salad.

176 calories per serving (4)
117 calories per serving (6)
Serves 4–6

300g potatoes, unpeeled and sliced into rounds
2 large courgettes, sliced into rounds
2 red onions, peeled and cut into thin wedges
2 peppers (red or green) cut into chunks
a few garlic cloves, unpeeled
1 tsp dried oregano or mixed herbs
1 tbsp olive oil
100ml white wine
300ml vegetable stock, chicken stock or water
12 cherry tomatoes
freshly ground black pepper

Preheat the oven to 200°C/Fan 180°C/Gas 6.

Put all the vegetables and garlic in a large roasting tin or shallow casserole dish. Sprinkle over the herbs and season well with black pepper. Drizzle over the olive oil, then mix everything together with your hands so all the vegetables have a coating of oil.

Mix the wine with the stock or water and pour over the vegetables. Either cover your roasting tin with foil or put the lid on your casserole dish, then place in the preheated oven for half an hour.

Remove the foil or lid and gently turn everything over with a spoon. Dot the cherry tomatoes around the dish, then put it back in the oven for another half an hour, uncovered, until most of the liquid has evaporated and the vegetables have started to brown.

RAINBOW VEGETABLE 'COUSCOUS'

This vegetable version of couscous tastes as awesome as it looks. And the good news is that you can have a nice big serving because it's low in calories.

114 calories per serving
Serves 4

¼ cauliflower
1 small head of broccoli
1 large carrot, cut into chunks
100g baby corn, roughly chopped
¼ red cabbage, shredded
½ red pepper
small bunch of parsley, coriander or mint, finely chopped
freshly ground black pepper

DRESSING (OPTIONAL)
1 tbsp olive oil
juice and zest of ½ lemon
juice of 1 orange
½ tsp ground cardamom

Divide the cauliflower and the broccoli into florets. One at a time, pulse the cauliflower, broccoli, carrot, corn and cabbage in a food processor until they resemble coarse breadcrumbs in texture. Be careful not to overprocess them as you don't want them to go mushy. Dice the red pepper as finely as possible.

Add water to a large frying pan – just enough to cover the base and no more than 100ml. Add all the vegetables and season them with pepper. Cook over a medium heat, stirring regularly, until the liquid has evaporated and the vegetables look fairly dry – this should take about 5 minutes.

Allow the vegetables to cool, then fluff them up a little and stir in the herbs. If you're serving the 'couscous' with a dish with a sauce you won't need a dressing, but this is also nice served on its own as a salad.

If adding the dressing, simply whisk the ingredients together and season with pepper. Add the dressing to the vegetable 'couscous' and serve.

HOME-MADE BAKED BEANS

Everyone loves baked beans and our home-made version is extra tasty while cutting down on the sugar. This is best made with dried beans that you've soaked overnight, but you can whip it up using a couple of cans if you're short of time. We like haricot beans, but you can use anything that takes your fancy. Check the packet for cooking times, though, if you do use different beans.

103 calories per serving
Serves 8 as a side dish

200g dried haricot or other beans (or 2 x 400g cans of
 cooked beans)
2 bay leaves
1 slice of onion
2 cloves
1 onion, very finely diced
1 carrot, very finely diced
1 celery stick, trimmed and very finely diced
1 tbsp vegetable oil
150ml vegetable stock
400g can of tomatoes
1 tbsp soy sauce
½ tsp sweet smoked paprika

pinch of ground cloves
freshly ground black pepper

If you're using dried beans, soak them overnight in plenty
of cold water. Drain the beans, then put them in a large
saucepan, add water to cover generously and bring to the boil.
Keep skimming off any foam that forms until it turns white.
Add the bay leaves, onion slice and cloves and continue to
boil for 10 minutes, then turn the heat down and simmer for
45–60 minutes. The beans should be cooked through but
not too soft, so check them regularly after 45 minutes. Drain,
discarding the cooking liquid, bay, onion and cloves.

Meanwhile, prepare the vegetables. They should be chopped
as finely as possible – almost to a purée – so you could use a
food processor. Heat the oil in a saucepan, add the vegetables
and cook them slowly for 10 minutes. Towards the end of
this time, turn up the heat slightly so the vegetables start to
caramelise – this adds sweetness to the sauce. Pour in the
stock and simmer for 5 minutes, then add the tomatoes, soy
sauce, paprika and cloves. Season with pepper and leave to
simmer for about half an hour until the sauce is well reduced.

Using a stick blender or ordinary blender, purée the sauce until
smooth. Tip it back into the pan, then add the beans (freshly
cooked or canned). Simmer for about 15 minutes to allow the
flavours to blend.

TOMATO SAUCE

This is a great basic tomato sauce to use with pasta or anything else. It's worth doubling up and making plenty, as it freezes well.

350 calories
Makes 1 quantity

---

1 tbsp olive oil

1 large onion, finely chopped

3 garlic cloves, finely chopped

2 x 400g cans of tomatoes

200ml red wine

1 tsp dried oregano

pinch of cinnamon

freshly ground black pepper

Heat the olive oil in a large saucepan. Add the onion and cook it very gently until it's soft and translucent, stirring regularly. Add the garlic and cook for another minute or so.

Add the tomatoes and wine, together with the dried oregano and cinnamon. Pour in 100ml of water, then season with pepper. Bring the sauce to the boil, then turn down the heat to a simmer and cover the pan. Cook for 30 minutes, then take the lid off the pan. The sauce can be used like this while it's quite thin, or you can cook it for longer, uncovered, until it has reduced and thickened.

This recipe can be varied to suit your taste – for example, swap red wine for white if you want a lighter, less robust sauce, or use some thyme or rosemary in place of oregano. The pinch of cinnamon works well, adding a hint of sweetness to offset any acidity in the tomatoes.

VEGETABLE STOCK

This is a good basic vegetable stock and it's great to have in your freezer to add flavour to soups, stews and other dishes.

1 tsp olive oil

2 large onions, roughly chopped

3 large carrots, well washed, chopped

200g squash or pumpkin, unpeeled, diced

4 celery sticks, sliced

2 leeks, sliced

100ml white wine or vermouth

1 large thyme sprig

1 large parsley sprig

1 bay leaf

a few peppercorns

Heat the olive oil in a large saucepan. Add all the vegetables and fry them over a high heat, stirring regularly, until they're starting to brown and caramelise around the edges. This will take at least 10 minutes. Add the white wine or vermouth and boil until it has evaporated away.

Cover the veg with 2 litres of water and add the herbs and peppercorns. Bring to the boil, then turn the heat down to a gentle simmer. Cook the stock, uncovered, for about an hour, stirring every so often.

Check the stock – the colour should have some depth to it. Strain it through a colander or a sieve lined with muslin, kitchen paper or coffee filter paper into a bowl and store it in the fridge for up to a week. Alternatively, pour the stock into freezer-proof containers and freeze.

CHICKEN STOCK

This is a great stock to make with your roast chicken carcass and if you like, you can save a few carcasses up in the freezer to make a larger quantity of stock. You can store the stock in the fridge for up to four days, or you can freeze it.

2 onions, unpeeled and quartered

2 carrots, roughly chopped

1 tbsp olive oil

1–3 chicken carcasses

1 thyme sprig

2 celery sticks, roughly chopped

a few peppercorns

1 bay leaf

parsley stems

Preheat the oven to its highest temperature. Put the onions and carrots in a roasting tin and drizzle them with the oil, then roast them until they are starting to char. Alternatively, you can do this in a pan on the hob. The idea is to caramelise the vegetables to enrich the stock.

Break the chicken carcasses up a little, then put them in a saucepan with the remaining ingredients and cover with water. Use up to a litre for one carcass and up to 1.5 litres for 2 or 3, but don't add so much water that the chicken is floating around. It needs to be quite a snug fit. Bring the water to the boil and skim off any mushroom-coloured foam that collects on top. Keep skimming until the foam turns white, then turn down the heat and cover the pan. Simmer the stock very gently for 1½–2 hours.

Strain the stock through a sieve lined with kitchen paper or muslin, but don't push the bits through if you want a clear stock. Discard all the solids. Leave the stock to cool to room temperature, then chill it in the fridge. When it is cold, you can remove any fat that's sitting on top.

BIKER TIP

You can reduce the stock down further to get a more concentrated flavour and freeze it in ice-cube trays. Once the cubes are frozen, turn them out into a plastic bag or container and store it in the freezer.

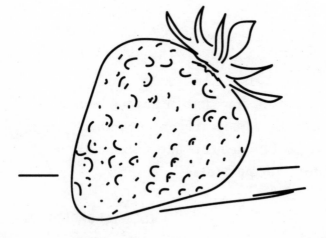

PUDDINGS
and
BAKES

7

Like most people, we both enjoy a little something sweet now and again. Unfortunately, most puddings and sweet treats are high in sugar and fat – so contain lots of calories – and are not a good idea if you have diabetes and you are trying to lose weight. It's best to stick with fresh fruit for dessert most of the time. But, for those moments when you feel like a change, we do have a few ideas that won't disrupt your diet too much and still taste scrumptious. You will also find that the less sugar you have the less you'll want, and your palate will soon adjust to food that is not so sweet.

Summer pudding 218

Coconut and carrot macaroons 222

Instant banana ice cream 224

Grilled pineapple 226

Sweet omelette 228

Aztec chocolate avocado mousse 232

Baked bananas with chocolate rum sauce 234

Ice lollies 236

Crunchy oat cookies 240

SUMMER PUDDING

There's virtually no fat in this traditional British dessert and if
you use good ripe fruit you don't need much sweetener either.
A large white sandwich loaf works a treat for the bread casing.
(*See photo on colour plate P.*)

131 calories per serving
Serves 6

---

low-cal oil spray

6 slices of white bread, crusts removed

300g strawberries, hulled and cut up if large

200g raspberries

200g blueberries

100g redcurrants, stalks removed, plus extra to garnish

sugar-free sweetener, to taste

Lightly spritz a 900ml pudding basin with oil, and line it with cling film. Take a slice of bread and cut it into a round that will fit into the bottom of the basin. Cut the rest of the slices into thirds widthways and use most of these to line the sides. Overlap them very slightly with one another and the base to ensure there are no gaps and press the bread down as much as possible. You should have a couple of slices left over to put on top of the fruit.

Put all the fruit in a saucepan and add 3 tablespoons of water. Simmer very gently until the fruit is lightly cooked and has given out a lot of juice. The liquid should be a deep reddish purple. Stir as little as possible to avoid breaking up the fruit too much. You will find that most of the raspberries will break up anyway but that's fine, as they will provide juice for the pudding. Taste for sweetness and add a little sweetener to get the flavour you like.

Ladle some of the fruit juice into the bottom of the basin and allow it to soak into the bread. Then with a slotted spoon, transfer all the fruit to the pudding basin. Pour in as much of the juice as possible, without it overflowing, then top with the remaining bread.

CONTINUED ON NEXT PAGE

Put a saucer on top of the pudding and weight it down with something heavy, such as a can of tomatoes. Put the pudding in the fridge and leave it for several hours, preferably overnight. Save any leftover juice for covering white patches and serving with the pudding.

When you are ready to serve, place a serving plate upside-down on top of the basin and turn the basin over to unmould the pudding. Carefully peel off the cling film. Cover any white patches with leftover fruit juice and garnish with extra berries if you have some.

Serve with dollops of low-fat crème fraiche, if you like, but don't forget to bear in mind the extra calories.

Raspberries and strawberries are not only delicious to eat but good for you too! They're rich in nutrients and fibre, but low in sugar, so a great choice if you have type 2 diabetes.

COCONUT AND CARROT MACAROONS

These are not the trendy French macaroons, but the old-fashioned sort, like our mams used to bake. We've cut back the calories by adding carrot and less coconut, so for once you can have your cake and eat it!

84 calories per macaroon
Makes 12

---

2 egg whites at room temperature

pinch of salt

60g caster sugar

100g carrot, finely grated

100g desiccated coconut

1 tsp vanilla extract

1 tbsp cornflour or plain flour

Preheat the oven to 180°C/Fan 160°C/Gas 4. Line a baking tray with baking paper or use a non-stick baking tray.

Whisk the egg whites with a pinch of salt until they form soft peaks – this should only take a couple of minutes. Then add all the sugar and continue to whisk until the mixture is shiny and full of air.

Squeeze out any excess liquid from the grated carrot and add it to the egg whites. Add the coconut and the vanilla extract, sift in the flour, then stir to mix everything together thoroughly. Be gentle so you don't lose all the air.

Put heaped tablespoons of the mixture at well-spaced intervals on the baking tray – you should get 12. Bake the macaroons in the oven for 15–20 minutes until golden brown. Remove them from the baking tray and leave them on a wire rack to cool.

INSTANT BANANA ICE CREAM

This sounds bonkers but it's brilliant. It's the speediest ice cream ever and tastes like a real treat, even though it contains very little fat and you can use sugar-free sweetener instead of sugar. All you need to do is think ahead and get the bananas into the freezer and then you can whip up a pud in no time. (*See photo on colour plate O.*)

100 calories per serving (4)
67 calories per serving (6)
Prep: 10 minutes (plus freezing time)
Serves 4–6

---

4 very ripe bananas
juice of ½ lime
grated zest of ½ lime, plus extra to garnish
½ tsp cinnamon, plus extra to garnish (optional)
a few drops of vanilla extract
calorie-free sweetener, to taste
100ml yoghurt or reduced-fat crème fraiche

Peel the bananas and cut them into fairly small chunks. Toss the chunks in the lime juice and arrange them on a baking tray. Put them in the freezer and leave them until they're completely solid all the way through – this will take at least 2 hours, but leave them overnight if possible.

Put the frozen bananas in a food processor with the lime zest, cinnamon, vanilla extract, sweetener and the yoghurt or crème fraiche. Blend until the mixture is beautifully thick, smooth and creamy, then serve sprinkled with some extra lime zest and cinnamon if you like.

GRILLED PINEAPPLE

If you're really in a hurry, you can buy pineapple ready cored and cut up. Otherwise it's no trouble to peel and core it yourself and the rest of the recipe takes minutes. This is one of our favourite desserts when we're trying to shed some timber. Tropically fantastic. (*See photo on colour plate O.*)

92 calories per serving (2 wedges)
Serves 4

8 wedges of peeled and cored pineapple (about 400g)
juice of 1 lime
1 tbsp maple syrup or runny honey
1 tsp ground ginger
1 tbsp rum (optional)
4 tbsp yoghurt or reduced-fat crème fraiche, to serve

Heat a griddle until it's very hot. This will take at least 5 minutes over a high heat. Put the pineapple wedges in a bowl.

While the griddle is heating, whisk the lime juice with the maple syrup or honey, ground ginger and rum, if using, in a small jug. Pour this over the pineapple wedges and mix thoroughly so they are all well coated – it's easiest to do this with your hands.

Remove the wedges of pineapple from the bowl, draining off and reserving any excess juices, and place them on the hot griddle. Grill for 2–3 minutes on each side until the pineapple is heated through and is marked with char lines.

Serve with yoghurt or crème fraiche and pour over any reserved juices.

SWEET OMELETTE

Everyone knows that an omelette is the perfect quick meal, but a sweet omelette also makes a good speedy pudding – a little bit of eggstacy! You can use any fruit you like for the compote or just serve the omelette with fresh fruit and crème fraiche. This makes one big omelette to share between two, but you could also make individual ones in smaller pans. Arrowroot is a bit like cornflour and is used for thickening dishes such as sauces. It's available in supermarkets. (*See photo on colour plate P.*)

217 calories per serving
Serves 2

---

2 large eggs
2 tsp caster sugar
low-cal olive oil spray or 2g butter
2 dessertspoons reduced-fat crème fraiche, to serve

QUICK FRUIT COMPOTE
150g blueberries or pitted black cherries (canned or jarred
    are fine)
zest and juice of ½ lime
1 tsp arrowroot
calorie-free sweetener, to taste

First make the compote. Put the blueberries or cherries in a saucepan with the lime zest and juice and add 2 tablespoons of water. Cook gently until the blueberries have softened.

Mix the arrowroot with a little cold water in a small bowl and stir until you have a completely smooth paste. Add this to the blueberries and stir until the sauce has thickened, then add sweetener to taste. Keep the compote warm while you make the omelette. Put the grill on at its highest setting to heat up.

Break the eggs into a bowl and add the sugar. Using a hand-held electric whisk, beat the eggs and sugar until they are full of air and you can trail a ribbon across the surface – this should take 3–4 minutes.

Spritz a non-stick frying pan with low-cal oil or melt the tiniest amount of butter and wipe it over the base of the pan so it is entirely covered. Tip the egg mixture into the frying pan, using a palette knife to make sure it covers the base evenly.

Cook the omelette over a medium heat for no longer than 2 minutes. To check the underside, lift up an edge – it should be just set and have a very light golden brown colour. Be careful when you do this, as the omelette is very delicate at this stage.

CONTINUED ON NEXT PAGE

Put the pan under the hot grill and cook the omelette until the top is also set and starting to brown very lightly. This will only take a couple of minutes so watch the omelette constantly to make sure you don't overcook it.

Remove the pan from the grill and gently fold the omelette in half, then cut it down the middle. Serve with the fruit compote and a little crème fraiche.

The less sugar you have, the less you will crave it. Good to know that things will get easier!

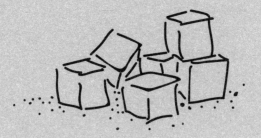

AZTEC CHOCOLATE AVOCADO MOUSSE

Dave first came across this treat in California – sounds weird but it really is good. It's simple and quick to make but success depends on using very ripe, creamy, non-fibrous avocados. Good Hass avocados are probably best. You need a jar of stem ginger in syrup and you could use some of the syrup in the mousse instead of honey.

247 calories per serving (6)
185 calories per serving (8)
Serves 6–8

---

2 avocados, peeled and roughly mashed
zest and juice of ½ lime
1 ball of stem ginger, roughly chopped
100g dark chocolate (70% cocoa solids)
50g honey (or syrup from the stem ginger)
100ml reduced-fat coconut milk
30g cocoa
1 tsp ground cinnamon
1 tsp ground ginger
¼ tsp ground allspice
¼ tsp ground cayenne

To serve

1 ball of stem ginger, finely sliced (optional)

Put the avocado, lime zest and juice and the piece of stem ginger in a food processor and blitz until fairly smooth – there might be a little texture from the stem ginger or lime zest.

Put the chocolate, honey or syrup, coconut milk, cocoa and spices in a small saucepan. Place the pan over a very gentle heat and whisk constantly until the chocolate has melted and you have a rich, dark mixture.

Scrape the chocolate mixture into the food processor with the avocado, lime and ginger and continue to blitz until everything is well combined and smooth.

Divide the mousse between 6 or 8 small glasses, espresso cups or bowls and chill until needed. Serve topped with some thin strips of stem ginger if you like.

BAKED BANANAS WITH CHOCOLATE RUM SAUCE

Well – chocolate rum sauce is not something you expect to find in a diet book, but we like to look after you all, and we do love something sweet from time to time. In fact, the sauce is made with only a small amount of dark chocolate and isn't as calorific as it sounds, although it still tastes wicked! (*See photo on colour plate P.*)

194 calories per serving
Serves 4

---

1 tsp butter

4 bananas

1 tsp demerara sugar

1 tbsp rum

CHOCOLATE RUM SAUCE

50g dark chocolate

50ml milk

1 tsp soft light brown sugar

1 tbsp rum

Preheat the oven to 200°C/Fan 180°C/Gas 6. Line a baking tray with a piece of foil that's big enough to overlap the edges of the tray slightly. Rub the foil with half the butter.

Peel the bananas and cut each one in half lengthways. Arrange the bananas on the foil and sprinkle over the sugar and rum. Take another piece of foil and rub it with the rest of the butter. Place the foil, buttered side down, over the bananas and crimp the edges of the pieces of foil together. Put the bananas in the oven and bake for 20 minutes.

Meanwhile, make the sauce. Break up the chocolate and put it in a saucepan with the milk, sugar and rum. Heat gently until the chocolate has melted, then whisk the sauce quite vigorously to make sure everything has combined properly. Remove the pan from the heat – the sauce will thicken slightly as it cools.

Take the bananas out of the oven and drizzle with spoonfuls of the chocolate sauce, then serve at once.

ICE LOLLIES

We made these in ice lolly trays with six holes, each holding about 50ml, but you can use any moulds you like – or even ice cube trays. Super refreshing on a hot summer day.

Pina colada ice lollies

Pineapples vary enormously in sweetness so you may or may not need to add sweetener to these.

34 calories per 50ml lolly

150ml reduced-fat coconut milk
150g fresh or canned pineapple
1 tbsp rum
calorie-free sweetener, to taste (optional)

Put the coconut milk, pineapple (drained, if using canned), and the rum in a blender and blitz until smooth. Taste for sweetness and add some sweetener if you think it needs it, then blitz again. Spoon off any foam and pour the liquid into moulds or ice cube trays and freeze until set.

Blueberry, banana and yoghurt ice lollies

35 calories per 50ml lolly

100ml fat-free natural yoghurt
1 banana (about 100g peeled weight)
juice of ½ lime
100g blueberries
a few drops of vanilla extract
calorie-free sweetener, to taste

Put the yoghurt, banana, lime juice and half the blueberries in a blender with the vanilla extract. Blend until fairly smooth. There'll probably still be some flecks of blueberry but that's fine. Add sweetener to taste.

Add the remaining blueberries and pulse a couple of times to break them up roughly. Pour into moulds or ice cube trays and freeze until set.

Strawberry and orange ice lollies

25 calories per 50ml lolly

200g strawberries
juice of 1–2 oranges (about 100ml)
juice of ½ lime
calorie-free sweetener, to taste

Put the berries and juice in a blender and blitz until smooth, then add sweetener to taste. If you want to get rid of the strawberry seeds, sieve the mixture before pouring it into your moulds or ice cube trays, then freeze until set.

We know that staying hydrated is so important for our health. We stick with water and avoid sweet fizzy drinks, which don't do you any good at all.

CRUNCHY OAT COOKIES

Some shop-bought cereal bars are scarily high in calories so try making these instead. At only 156 calories each, our cookies make a tasty little morsel with a cuppa. The oats fill you up and keep you going too. (*See photo on colour plate O.*)

156 calories per cookie
Makes about 16

100g plain flour

1 tsp baking powder

pinch of salt

200g porridge oats

75g raisins

85g butter, softened

100g light brown sugar

1 egg, beaten

Preheat the oven to 180°C/Fan 160°C/Gas 4.

Put the flour in a bowl with the baking powder and a pinch of salt. Whisk briefly to make sure there aren't any lumps, then stir in the porridge oats and raisins.

Put the butter and sugar in a separate bowl and whisk until very light and fluffy. Beat in the egg, then combine the butter mixture with the dry ingredients. Mix thoroughly.

Take tablespoons of the mixture, forming them into little balls about the size of a ping-pong ball, and place them on a baking tray. Flatten the balls down a little so they aren't too thick in the middle.

Bake the cookies in the oven for 12–15 minutes until lightly coloured. Remove them from the oven and leave them to set on the baking tray for 3 minutes, before transferring them to a rack to cool.

MEAL PLANNERS

Just to help you get started, we've put together some ideas for weekly menus – two weeks of general plans for meat and fish eaters, and two weeks for vegetarians. The calorie counts for each day work out to roughly 1,500 calories: that is about 300 for breakfast, 400 for lunch and 600 for the evening meal, plus two snacks of about 100 calories. We've also allowed for 150ml of semi-skimmed milk a day for your tea and coffee. Feel free to swap to different dishes, but try to keep the calorie count about the same. And if you don't have time to cook every day, try making a big batch of soup or salad at the start of the week and enjoy it for a few days. Whatever suits you. Also, it's always a good idea to add extra veg to any of the main dishes – have a look at the recipes in the Sides and Basics chapter, or have some steamed broccoli, spinach or other greens. Drink plenty of water and – very important – check with your doctor before starting on a diet.

GENERAL PLAN

WEEK ONE

MONDAY

Breakfast
2 boiled eggs + 2 slices wholemeal toast with 1 tsp olive oil spread

Snack
1 medium orange

Lunch
Chunky chicken soup (p.54) + 1 wholemeal roll (60g)

Snack
1 oatcake + Salsa (p.88) + red pepper and carrot sticks

Evening meal
Caribbean chicken curry (p.174) + 50g (uncooked weight) brown rice

Pudding
1 medium apple

TUESDAY

Breakfast
Avocado on toast (p.22)

Snack
1 medium banana

Lunch
Smoked trout salad (p.68) + 1 wholemeal roll (60g) with 1 tsp olive oil spread

Snack
2 tbsp (30g) reduced-fat hummus + red pepper and carrot sticks

Evening meal
Roast vegetable lasagne, with dried pasta (p.110) + mixed salad with 2 tsp dressing

Pudding
Grilled pineapple (p.226)

WEDNESDAY

Breakfast
1 small pot low-fat yoghurt + 40g sugar-free muesli

Snack
1 pear

Lunch
Roast chicken breast +
Tabbouleh (p.62)

Snack
1 rye cracker + Carrot, red
pepper and butter bean dip
(p.78)

Evening meal
2 White bean and tuna
fishcakes (p.144) + 1 baked
sweet potato (200g) +
5 tbsp tzatziki

Pudding
1 medium orange

THURSDAY

Breakfast
Stove-top granola (p.16) +
150ml semi-skimmed milk +
1 small (80g) banana

Snack
1 small pot low-fat yoghurt

Lunch
Lunch-box noodles (p.76)

Snack
1–2 rye crispbreads with 20g
peanut butter

Evening meal
Barley risotto with greens –
with cheese (p.100)

Pudding
100g fresh pineapple

FRIDAY

Breakfast
Porridge with raspberries

Snack
2 medium kiwis

Lunch
Smoked haddock omelette
(p.26) + green salad with
2 tsp dressing

Snack
20g almonds

Evening meal
Chilli prawn pasta (p.162)

Pudding
1 small pot low-fat yoghurt

SATURDAY

Breakfast
Avocado on toast (p.22)

Snack
1 hard-boiled egg

Lunch
Bean and vegetable soup
(p.50) + 1 wholemeal roll
with 1 tsp olive oil spread

Snack
1 medium orange

Evening meal
Lamb dhansak (p.182) +
50g (uncooked weight)
brown rice

Pudding
Instant banana ice cream
(p.224)

SUNDAY

Breakfast
Buckwheat pancakes with
eggs and mushrooms (p.32)

Snack
Crunchy oat cookie (p.240)

Lunch
Pea, lettuce and asparagus
soup (p.44) + 1 wholemeal
roll with 1 tsp olive oil spread

Snack
Roast chickpeas (p.90)

Evening meal
Chicken tray bake with fennel,
peas and new potatoes
(p.172)

Pudding
Aztec chocolate avocado
mousse (p.232)

WEEK TWO

MONDAY

Breakfast
Stove-top granola (p.16) +
150ml semi-skimmed milk
+ 1 small (80g) banana

Snack
80g pomegranate

Lunch
Quick Mexican eggs (p.30)

Snack
Almonds (20g)

Evening meal
Fish crumble (p.158)

Pudding
Coconut and carrot macaroon
(p.222)

TUESDAY

Breakfast
2 boiled eggs + 2 slices
wholemeal toast with 1 tsp
olive oil spread

Snack
1 small pot low-fat yoghurt

Lunch
Tomato soup (p.42) +
wholemeal roll

Snack
1–2 rye crackers, each spread
with 1 tbsp (15g) light soft
cheese)

Evening meal
Beef stir-fry (p.180) +
150g straight to wok noodles

Pudding
Half a small mango (100g)

WEDNESDAY

Breakfast
Apple and oat smoothie
(p.18)

Snack
1 medium banana

Lunch
Harissa vegetables with
jumbo couscous (p.64) +
100g cooked peeled prawns
+ 5 tbsp tzatziki

Snack
Spiced popcorn (p.92)

Evening meal
Fish curry (p.150) +
50g (uncooked weight)
brown rice

Pudding
1 small pot low-fat yoghurt

THURSDAY

Breakfast
Half grapefruit + scrambled
eggs (2 medium eggs,
1 tsp butter) + 1 slice
wholemeal toast

Snack
2 medium kiwis

Lunch
Chicken breast + Summery
green coleslaw (p.60)

Snack
1 rye cracker + Smoked
trout dip (p.80)

Evening meal
Salmon and broccoli tray
bake (p.152) + 3 new potatoes

Pudding
1 medium banana

FRIDAY

Breakfast
3 heaped tbsp muesli +
150ml semi-skimmed milk,
handful of raspberries

Snack
Banana, strawberry and
blueberry smoothie (p.20)

Lunch
Scotch broth (p.56) +
wholemeal roll and 1 tsp
olive oil spread

Snack
50g hummus + sticks of raw
vegetables

Evening meal
Latin American shepherd's
pie (p.122)

Pudding
Grilled pineapple (p.226)

SATURDAY

Breakfast
Mediterranean Biker brunch
(p.28) + 1 slice wholemeal
toast with 1 tsp olive oil
spread and 2 tsp reduced-
sugar jam or marmalade

Snack
1 medium apple

Lunch
Tuna and caper wrap (p.82)
+ 1 small pot low-fat yoghurt

Snack
Spiced popcorn (p.92)

Evening meal
Garlic chicken with beans,
kale and cherry tomatoes
(p.168)

Pudding
Baked bananas with
chocolate rum sauce (p.234)

Evening meal
Pork souvlaki with light salsa
verde (p.184)

Pudding
Summer pudding (p.218)

SUNDAY

Breakfast
Corned beef hash (p.36)

Snack
1 medium banana

Lunch
Smoked trout salad (p.68)
+ wholemeal roll with 1 tsp
olive oil spread

Snack
Tuna and caper dip (p.82) +
1–2 rye crackers

VEGETARIAN PLAN

WEEK ONE

MONDAY

Breakfast
1 small pot low-fat yoghurt +
40g sugar-free muesli

Snack
1 medium orange

Lunch
Pesto-stuffed mushrooms
(p.128) + wholemeal roll with 1
tsp olive oil spread

Snack
20g almonds

Evening meal
Vegetable curry (p.114) +
75g (uncooked weight)
brown rice + 5 tbsp tzatziki

Pudding
Ice lolly (p.236)

TUESDAY

Breakfast
Stove-top granola (p.16) +
150ml semi-skimmed milk

Snack
20g almonds

Lunch
Grilled aubergines with
chickpea and spinach salad
(p.134) + wholemeal roll and
1 tsp olive oil spread

Snack
1 medium banana

Evening meal
Black-eyed beans and greens
(p.116) + 75g (uncooked
weight) brown rice

Pudding
1 medium apple

WEDNESDAY

Breakfast
2 slices wholemeal bread
with 2 tsp olive oil spread and
2 tsp reduced-sugar jam

Snack
1 medium banana

Lunch
Bean and vegetable soup
(p.50) + wholemeal roll and
1 tsp olive oil spread

Snack
Crunchy oat cookie (p.240)

Evening meal
Vegetarian pasta (p.118)

Pudding
I small pot low-fat yoghurt

THURSDAY

Breakfast
Porridge + handful of
blueberries

Snack
1 medium apple

Lunch
Red lentil and harissa soup
(p.48) + 1 wholemeal roll and
1 tsp olive oil spread

Snack
20g almonds

Evening meal
Roast vegetable lasagne, with
dried pasta (p.110) + mixed
salad with 2 tsp dressing

Pudding
Half a small mango (100g)

FRIDAY

Breakfast
Apple and oat smoothie
(p.18)

Snack
20g almonds

Lunch
Lunch-box pot noodles (p.76)

Snack
Roast chickpeas (p.90)

Evening meal
Barley risotto with greens,
with cheese (p.100)

Pudding
Summer pudding (p.218)

SATURDAY

Breakfast
Quick Mexican eggs (p.30)

Snack
Green smoothie (p.19)

Lunch
Tomato soup (p.42) +
wholemeal roll

Snack
Crunchy oat cookie (p.240)

Evening meal
Latin American shepherd's
pie (p.122)

Pudding
Aztec chocolate avocado
mousse (p.232)

SUNDAY

Breakfast
3 heaped tbsp muesli +
150ml semi-skimmed milk
+ handful of blueberries

Snack
1–2 oatcakes spread with
reduced-sugar jam

Lunch
Bean and vegetable soup
(p.50) + 1 wholemeal roll and
1 tsp olive oil spread

Snack
1 small pot low-fat yoghurt

Evening meal
Baked potatoes with broccoli
and cheese (p.98) +
Home-made baked beans
(p.206)

Pudding
Baked banana with chocolate
rum sauce (p.234)

WEEK TWO

MONDAY

Breakfast
2 slices wholemeal toast
with 2 tsp peanut butter +
1 banana

Snack
1 medium apple

Lunch
Harissa vegetables and
jumbo couscous (p.64) +
5 tbsp guacamole

Snack
1–2 rye crackers plus carrot,
red pepper, and butter bean
dip (p.78)

Evening meal
Vegetarian pasta (p.118) +
mixed green salad with
1 tbsp dressing

Pudding
1 small pot low-fat yoghurt

TUESDAY

Breakfast
Porridge + handful of
blueberries

Snack
1 medium orange

Lunch
Hummus salad wrap, made
with 60g hummus, 1 large
wholemeal wrap and salad

Snack
20g almonds

Evening meal
Cauliflower and broccoli
cheese (p.126) + Spring
greens with harissa and
garlic (p.198)

Pudding
Half a small mango (100g)

WEDNESDAY

Breakfast
Half grapefruit + scrambled
eggs (2 medium eggs,
1 tsp butter) + 1 slice
wholemeal toast

Snack
1 small pot low-fat yoghurt

Lunch
Courgette, mint and lemon
soup (p.46) + 1 wholemeal
roll + 40g veggie Cheddar

Snack
Lil's roast vegetable dip
(p.86) + raw red pepper
and carrot sticks

Evening meal
Latin American shepherd's
pie (p.122)

Pudding
Grilled pineapple (p.226)

THURSDAY

Breakfast
1 small pot low-fat yoghurt +
1 medium banana +
2 tbsp sugar-free muesli

Snack
1 medium pear

Lunch
Roast carrot, pepper
and chickpea salad (p.58)
+ 1 medium (150g) avocado

Snack
1–2 rye crispbreads +
Carrot, red pepper and butter
bean dip (p.78)

Evening meal
Roast vegetable lasagne
(p.110)

Pudding
Instant banana ice cream
(p.224)

FRIDAY

Breakfast
Avocado on toast (p.22)

Snack
2 kiwis

Lunch
Vegetable frittata (p.24) +
3 small new potatoes +
green salad with 2 tsp
dressing

Snack
1–2 oatcakes each spread
with 1 tbsp Salsa (p.88)

Evening meal
Barley risotto with greens,
with cheese (p.100)

Pudding
1 small pot low-fat yoghurt

SATURDAY

Breakfast
Buckwheat pancakes with
eggs and mushrooms (p.32)

Snack
Banana, strawberry and
blueberry smoothie (p.20)

Lunch
Rainbow vegetable
'couscous' (p.204) + half
an avocado

Snack
50g olives + 2 breadsticks

Evening meal
Thai vegetable curry (p.102)
+ 75g (uncooked weight)
brown rice

Pudding
Summer pudding (p.218)

SUNDAY

Breakfast
Apple and oat smoothie
(p.18)

Snack
Crunchy oat cookie (p.240)

Lunch
Red lentil and harissa soup
(p.48) + 1 wholemeal roll with
1 tsp olive oil spread

Snack
1 small pot low-fat yoghurt

Evening meal
Aubergine bake with 2 balls
of mozzarella (p.106) + Root
vegetable boulangère (p.196)

Pudding
Sweet omelette (p.228)

INDEX

Figures in **bold** refer
to recipes that are
illustrated in the colour
sections.

almonds
  Stove-top granola
    16—17
apples
  Apple and oat
    smoothie **18**
  Green smoothie **19**
  Red cabbage with
    apple and chestnuts
    194—5
  Root vegetable rösti
    200—1
  Summery green
    coleslaw **60—61**
Artichoke and lemon
  dip **84—5**
asparagus
  Pea, lettuce and
    asparagus soup
    44—5
aubergines 109
  Aubergine bake
    106—8
  Grilled aubergines
    with chickpea and
    spinach salad
    134—6
  Lil's roast vegetable
    dip **86—7**
  Roast vegetable
    lasagne 110—12
  Thai vegetable curry
    102—4

avocados 6
  Avocado on toast
    22—3
  Aztec chocolate
    avocado mousse
    232—3
  Chicken, squash and
    quinoa salad 70—71
  Salsa 30, 31
Aztec chocolate
  avocado mousse 232—3

bacon
  Bean and vegetable
    soup **50-52**
  Baked beans, Home-
    made 206—7
  Baked potatoes with
    broccoli and cheese
    98—9
bananas
  Baked bananas with
    chocolate rum sauce
    234—5
  Banana, strawberry
    and blueberry
    smoothie **20**
  Blueberry, banana and
    yoghurt ice lollies
    237
  Instant banana ice
    cream **224—5**
barley, pearl
  Barley risotto with
    greens **100—1**
  Scotch broth **56—7**
Bean and vegetable
  soup **50—52**

Béchamel sauce 110—11,
  112
Beef stir-fry **180—81**
beetroot
  Root vegetable rösti
    200—1
  Smoked trout salad
    68—9
  Smoked trout
    sandwich or wrap
    80—81
black beans
  Quick Mexican eggs
    30—31
black-eyed beans
(peas)
  Black-eyed beans
    and greens
    116—17
  Turkey chilli with
    cauliflower 'rice'
    164—6
blueberries
  Banana, strawberry
    and blueberry
    smoothie **20**
  Blueberry, banana and
    yoghurt ice lollies
    237
  Quick fruit compote
    228—9, 230
  Summer pudding
    218—20
broad beans
  Barley risotto with
    greens **100—1**
  Summery green
    coleslaw **60—61**

Vegetarian pasta
118—19
broccoli 9
Baked potatoes with
broccoli and cheese
98—9
Barley risotto with
greens **100—1**
Cauliflower and
broccoli cheese
126—7
Rainbow vegetable
'couscous' 204—5
Salmon and broccoli
tray bake **152—3**
Vegetable frittata
24—5
Bubble and squeak
130—32
Buckwheat pancakes
with eggs and
mushrooms **32—4**
bulgur wheat
Tabbouleh 62—3
butter beans
Carrot, red pepper
and butter bean dip
78—9
Latin American
shepherd's pie
122—4
Pesto-stuffed
mushrooms **128—9**
butternut squash
Chicken, squash and
quinoa salad 70—71
Lamb dhansak **182—3**
Roast vegetable
lasagne 110—12
Thai vegetable curry
102—4
Tomato soup **42—3**
Vegetable frittata
24—5
Vegetable stock
210—11

cabbage 9
Bean and vegetable
soup **50—52**

Bubble and squeak
130—32
Scotch broth **56—7**
Summery green
coleslaw **60—61**
cabbage, red
Rainbow vegetable
'couscous' 204—5
Red cabbage with
apple and chestnuts
194—5
cannellini beans
Bean and vegetable
soup **50—52**
Garlic chicken with
beans, kale and
cherry tomatoes
168—9
White bean and tuna
fishcakes 144—6
capers
Salsa verde 185, 186
Tuna and caper dip or
filling 82—3
Caribbean chicken
curry **174—6**
carrots 9
Bean and vegetable
soup **50-52**
Bubble and squeak
130—32
Carrot, red pepper
and butter bean dip
78—9
Chicken stock 212—13
Chunky chicken soup
54—5
Coconut and carrot
macaroons 222—3
Corned beef hash
36—7
Latin American
shepherd's pie 122—4
Lunch-box pot
noodles 76—7
Rainbow vegetable
'couscous' 204—5
Roasted carrot,
pepper and chickpea
salad **58—9**

Root vegetable
boulangère 196—7
Scotch broth **56—7**
Tomato soup **42—3**
Vegetable stock
210—11
cauliflower 9, 167
Cauliflower and
broccoli cheese
126—7
Cauliflower 'rice' 165,
166
Rainbow vegetable
'couscous' 204—5
Roast spiced
cauliflower 192—3
Thai vegetable curry
102—4
celeriac
Corned beef hash
36—7
Root vegetable rösti
200—1
Smoked trout salad
68—9
Tabbouleh 62—3
Tomato soup **42—3**
cheese 6
Baked potatoes with
broccoli and cheese
98—9
Cauliflower and
broccoli cheese
126—7
cherries
Quick fruit compote
228—9, 230
chestnuts
Red cabbage with
apple and chestnuts
194—5
chicken 10, 12, 140
Caribbean chicken
curry **174—6**
Chicken, squash and
quinoa salad 70—71
Chicken stock 212—13
Chicken tray bake
with fennel, peas and
new potatoes 172—3

Chunky chicken soup
54—5
Fusion tandoori
chicken 170—71
Garlic chicken with
beans, kale and
cherry tomatoes
168—9
Lunch-box pot
noodles 76—7
see also Turkey keema
peas
chickpeas
Grilled aubergines
with chickpea and
spinach salad 134—6
Roast chickpeas
90—91
Roasted carrot,
pepper and chickpea
salad **58—9**
Chilli prawn pasta **162—3**
chocolate 6
Aztec chocolate
avocado mousse
232—3
Baked bananas with
chocolate rum sauce
234—5
Chunky chicken soup
54—5
Coconut and carrot
macaroons 222—3
cod
Fish crumble **158—60**
coleslaw
Summery green
coleslaw **60—61**
Corned beef hash **36—7**
courgettes 9
Bean and vegetable
soup **50—52**
Courgette, mint and
lemon soup **46—7**
Greek-style roast
vegetables 202—3
Green pasta **120—21**
Harissa vegetables
and jumbo couscous
64—6

Lunch-box pot
noodles 76—7
Pesto-stuffed
mushrooms **128—9**
Summery green
coleslaw **60—61**
Tabbouleh 62—3
Thai vegetable curry
102—4
Vegetable curry
114—15
Vegetable frittata
24—5
Vegetarian pasta
118—19
couscous
Couscous topping
(for Fish crumble)
159, 160
Harissa vegetables
and jumbo couscous
64—6
Crunchy oat cookies
240—41
curries
Caribbean chicken
curry **174—6**
Fish curry **150—51**
Lamb dhansak **182—3**
Thai vegetable curry
102—4
Vegetable curry **114—15**

Dhansak, Lamb **182—3**
dips
Artichoke and lemon
dip **84—5**
Carrot, red pepper
and butter bean dip
78—9
Lil's roast vegetable
dip **86—7**
Smoked trout dip
80—81
Tuna and caper dip
82—3

eggs 3, 10, 12, 14, 133
Bubble and squeak
130—32

Buckwheat pancakes
with eggs and
mushrooms **32—4**
Coconut and carrot
macaroons 222—3
Corned beef hash
36—7
Mediterranean Biker
brunch **28—9**
Quick Mexican eggs
30—31
Smoked haddock
omelette 26—7
Sweet omelette
228—30
Vegetable frittata
24—5

fennel
Bean and vegetable
soup **50—52**
Chicken tray bake
with fennel, peas and
new potatoes 172—3
Mediterranean Biker
brunch **28—9**
Mediterranean fish
casserole **148—9**
Summery green
coleslaw **60—61**
fish 6, 10, 140, 147, 157
Baked fish with
red peppers and
tomatoes 142—3
Fish crumble **158—60**
Fish curry **150—51**
Mackerel fillets with
gremolata **154—6**
Mediterranean fish
casserole **148—9**
Salmon and broccoli
tray bake **152—3**
Smoked haddock
omelette 26—7
Smoked trout dip or
filling **80—81**
Smoked trout salad
68—9
Tuna and caper dip or
filling **82—3**

White bean and tuna
fishcakes 144—6
Frittata, Vegetable
24—5
Fusion tandoori chicken
170—71

Garlic chicken with
beans, kale and
cherry tomatoes
168—9
Granola, Stove-top
16—17
Greek-style roast
vegetables 202—3
Green pasta **120—21**
Gremolata **154, 155**

haddock, smoked
Fish crumble **158—60**
Smoked haddock
omelette 26—7
hake
Fish crumble
158—60
Fish curry **150—51**
haricot beans
Home-made baked
beans 206—7
harissa
Harissa vegetables
and jumbo couscous
64—6
Red lentil and harissa
soup **48—9**
Spring greens with
harissa and garlic
198—9
Home-made baked
beans 206—7

ice cream
Instant banana ice
cream **224—5**
ice lollies 236
Blueberry, banana and
yoghurt ice lollies
237
Pina colada ice lollies
236

Strawberry and
orange ice lollies 238
Instant banana ice
cream **224—5**

kale
Chunky chicken soup
54—5
Garlic chicken with
beans, kale and
cherry tomatoes
168—9
kidney beans
Latin American
shepherd's pie 122—4
Turkey chilli with
cauliflower 'rice'
164—6

lamb
Lamb dhansak **182—3**
Scotch broth **56—7**
lasagne
Roast vegetable
lasagne 110—12
Latin American
shepherd's pie 122—4
leeks
Pea, lettuce and
asparagus soup
44—5
Roast vegetable
lasagne 110—12
Scotch broth **56—7**
Tomato soup **42—3**
Vegetable stock
210—11
lentils
Lamb dhansak 182—3
Red lentil and harissa
soup **48-9**
Tomato soup **42—3**
Lil's roast vegetable dip
86—7
Lunch-box pot noodles
76—7

macaroons
Coconut and carrot
macaroons 222—3

Mackerel fillets with
gremolata **154—6**
Mediterranean Biker
brunch **28—9**
Mediterranean fish
casserole **148—9**
mousse
Aztec chocolate
avocado mousse
232—3
mushrooms 35
Beef stir-fry **180—81**
Buckwheat pancakes
with eggs and
mushrooms **32—4**
Lunch-box pot
noodles 76—7
Pesto-stuffed
mushrooms **128—9**
Salmon and broccoli
tray bake **152—3**
Vegetable curry
114—15

noodles
Lunch-box pot
noodles 76—7

oats
Apple and oat
smoothie **18**
Crunchy oat cookies
240—41
Stove-top granola
16—17
oranges 6—7
Green smoothie **19**
Strawberry and
orange ice lollies
238

pak choi
Beef stir-fry **180—81**
pancakes
Buckwheat pancakes
with eggs and
mushrooms **32—4**
parsnips
Root vegetable
boulangère 196—7

Root vegetable rösti
200—1
pasta
Bean and vegetable
soup **50—52**
Chilli prawn pasta
162—3
Green pasta **120—21**
Roast vegetable
lasagne 110—12
Vegetarian pasta
118—19
peas 9
Barley risotto with
greens **100—1**
Courgette, mint and
lemon soup **46—7**
Lunch-box pot
noodles 76—7
Pea, lettuce and
asparagus soup
44—5
Summery green
coleslaw **60—61**
peas, split
Scotch broth **56—7**
peppers 9
Baked fish with
red peppers and
tomatoes 142—3
Beef stir-fry **180—81**
Black-eyed beans
(peas) and greens
116—17
Carrot, red pepper
and butter bean dip
78—9
Chilli prawn pasta
162—3
Greek-style roast
vegetables 202—3
Harissa vegetables
and jumbo couscous
64—6
Latin American
shepherd's pie 122—4
Lil's roast vegetable
dip **86—7**
Lunch-box pot
noodles 76—7

Mediterranean Biker
brunch **28—9**
Mediterranean fish
casserole **148—9**
Rainbow vegetable
'couscous' 204—5
Roast vegetable
lasagne 110—12
Roasted carrot,
pepper and chickpea
salad **58—9**
Salmon and broccoli
tray bake **152—3**
Tabbouleh 62—3
Turkey chilli with
cauliflower 'rice'
164—6
Vegetable frittata
24—5
Pesto-stuffed
mushrooms **128—9**
Pina colada ice lollies
236
pineapple
Caribbean chicken
curry **174—6**
Grilled pineapple
226—7
Pina colada ice lollies
236
Popcorn, Spiced **92—3**
Pork souvlaki with light
salsa verde **184—6**
potatoes
Baked potatoes with
broccoli and cheese
98—9
Bubble and squeak
130—32
Caribbean chicken
curry **174—6**
Chicken tray bake
with fennel, peas and
new potatoes 172—3
Greek-style roast
vegetables 202—3
Mediterranean fish
casserole **148—9**
Root vegetable
boulangère 196—7

Root vegetable rösti
200—1
Salmon and broccoli
tray bake **152—3**
potatoes, sweet
Baked potatoes with
broccoli and cheese
98—9
Chunky chicken soup
54—5
prawns
Chilli prawn pasta
162—3
pumpkin
Caribbean chicken
curry **174—6**
Roast vegetable
lasagne 110—12
Vegetable stock
210—11

Quick fruit compote
228—9, 230
Quick Mexican eggs
30—31
quinoa
Chicken, squash and
quinoa salad 70—71

Rainbow vegetable
'couscous' 204—5
raspberries 221
Summer pudding
218—20
red cabbage *see*
cabbage, red
redcurrants
Summer pudding
218—20
Red lentil and harissa
soup **48—9**
risotto
Barley risotto with
greens **100—1**
Roast vegetable
lasagne 110—12
Root vegetable
boulangère 196—7
Root vegetable rösti
200—1

salads
  Chicken, squash and
    quinoa salad 70—71
  Chickpea and spinach
    salad 134—6
  Harissa vegetables
    and jumbo couscous
    64—6
  Roasted carrot,
    pepper and chickpea
    salad **58—9**
  Smoked trout salad
    68—9
  Summery green
    coleslaw **60—61**
  Tabbouleh 62—3
  Tomato and onion
    salad 154—5, 156
salmon 140
  Salmon and broccoli
    tray bake **152—3**
Salsa 30, 31
  Salsa verde 185, 186
  Socca and salsa **88—9**
sauces
  Béchamel sauce
    110—11, 112
  Chocolate rum sauce
    234, 235
  Tomato sauce 113,
    208—9
Scotch broth **56—7**
smoothies 21
  Apple and oat
    smoothie **18**
  Banana, strawberry
    and blueberry
    smoothie **20**
  Green smoothie **19**
Socca and salsa **88—9**
soups 40
  Bean and vegetable
    soup 50—52
  Chunky chicken soup
    54—5
  Courgette, mint and
    lemon soup 46—7
  Pea, lettuce and
    asparagus soup
    44—5

Red lentil and harissa
  soup 48—9
Scotch broth **56—7**
Tomato soup 42—3
spaghetti
  Chilli prawn pasta
    162—3
Spiced popcorn
  92—3
spinach 9
  Courgette, mint and
    lemon soup **46—7**
  Green smoothie **19**
  Grilled aubergines
    with chickpea and
    spinach salad
    134—6
  Pesto-stuffed
    mushrooms **128—9**
spring greens
  Black-eyed beans
    (peas) and greens
    116—17
  Spring greens with
    harissa and garlic
    198—9
squash see butternut
  squash
stir-fry
  Beef **180—81**
stocks 12
  Chicken stock 212—13
  Vegetable stock
    210—11
strawberries 221
  Banana, strawberry
    and blueberry
    smoothie **20**
  Strawberry and
    orange ice lollies
    238
  Summer pudding
    218—20
Summer pudding
  218—20
Summery green
  coleslaw **60—61**
swede
  Bubble and squeak
    130—32

Scotch broth **56—7**
sweetcorn 9
  Latin American
    shepherd's pie
    122—4

Tabbouleh 62—3
Thai vegetable curry
  102—4
Tomato and onion salad
  154—5, 156
Tomato sauce 113,
  208—9
Tomato soup **42—3**
tray bakes
  Chicken tray bake
    with fennel, peas and
    new potatoes 172—3
  Salmon and broccoli
    tray bake **152—3**
trout, smoked
  Smoked trout dip or
    filling **80—81**
  Smoked trout salad
    68—9
tuna
  Tuna and caper dip or
    filling **82—3**
  White bean and tuna
    fishcakes 144—6
turkey 140
  Turkey chilli with
    cauliflower 'rice'
    164—6
  Turkey keema peas
    178—9
turnips
  Scotch broth **56—7**

Vegetable curry **114—15**
Vegetable frittata 24—5
Vegetable stock 210—11
Vegetarian pasta
  118—19

White bean and tuna
  fishcakes 144—6

USEFUL ADDRESSES

UK

Diabetes UK Central Office

Wells Lawrence House

126 Back Church Lane

London E1 1FH

Phone: 0345 123 2399, or in Scotland, call 0141 212 8710

www.diabetes.org.uk

NHS - for general advice on diabetes

www.NHS.uk

Diabetes Research & Wellness Foundation

Building 6000

Langstone Technology Park

Havant

Hampshire, PO9 1SA

Phone: 023 92 637808

www.drwf.org.uk

IRELAND

Diabetes Ireland

19 Northwood House

Northwood Business Campus

Santry, Dublin 9

DO9 DH30

Phone: 01 842 8118

Email: info@diabetes.ie

www.diabetes.ie

AUSTRALIA
Australian Diabetes Society

145 Macquarie Street

Sydney, NSW 2000

Phone: 61-2-9169 3859

Email: admin@diabetessociety.com.au

www.diabetessociety.com.au

National Diabetes Services Scheme

GPO Box 9824

(in your state/territory capital city)

NDSS Helpline: 1800 637 700

www.ndss.com.au

Email: ndss@diabetesaustralia.com.au

NEW ZEALAND
Diabetes New Zealand

Level 10, 15 Murphy Street

Wellington, 6011

Phone toll-free: 0800 DIABETES (0800 342 238)

www.diabetes.org.nz

THANKS GANG

A big thank you to all our great team who helped us put this book together. As always, massive appreciation to Catherine Phipps, our recipe consultant, for her amazing foodie wisdom, and to Andrew Hayes-Watkins for the great photographs.

Thank you to Fiona Hunter, our nutrition and diet expert, and to Jinny Johnson, editor, for all their advice and assistance in creating this book, to Vicky Eribo at Orion for her guiding hand, and to Clare Sivell for the very elegant design. And we'd like to thank Lucie Stericker for the witty little illustrations.

Thank you to our wonderful food stylists – Anna Burges-Lumsden, Lisa Harrison and Mima Sinclair – for making the dishes for the photographs, and to Elise See Tai for proofreading and Vicki Robinson for the index.

Also, mega thanks to Professor Roy Taylor for all his help and advice in the past and for writing the foreword to this book.

Love and thanks to Amanda Harris, Natalie Zietcer and Emily Arthur at YMU.